How
Self-D

–
to Exercise

Practical Techniques
and Strategies to
Develop a Lifetime
Habit of Exercise

By Martin Meadows

Download another Book for Free

I want to thank you for buying my book and offer you another book (just as valuable as this book), *Grit: How to Keep Going When You Want to Give Up*, completely free.

Visit the link below to receive it:

http://www.profoundselfimprovement.com/selfdisciplinetoexercise

In *Grit*, I'll share with you exactly how to stick to your goals according to peak performers and science.

In addition to getting *Grit*, you'll also have an opportunity to get my new books for free, enter giveaways, and receive other valuable emails from me.

Again, here's the link to sign up:

http://www.profoundselfimprovement.com/selfdisciplinetoexercise

Table of Contents

Prologue

Imagine there's a pill that improves your ability to resist temptations and persevere. Your life is now so much better because it's so much easier to achieve your goals. The pill also provides other benefits like:

- a significant decrease in perceived stress and emotional distress,

- reduced smoking, alcohol and caffeine consumption,

- an increase in healthy eating,

- improved emotional control,

- an increase in attendance to commitments and maintenance of household chores,

- an increase in monitoring of spending,

- an improvement in study habits.

There are no side effects, and it's vastly available everywhere you go for free or a very low price. How many pills would you like to order today if such a pill existed?

Well, it actually does exist, though not in pill form. It's called *exercise*. All of the benefits listed above come from a 2006 Australian study on 24 non-exercisers between 18 and 50 who regularly exercised for a 2-month period (just once a week for the first month and three times a week for the second month)[i], and it's just one out of hundreds, if not thousands, of studies exploring the positive effects of exercise.

There's no question that regular physical activity is not an option – it's a necessity for both your mind and your body.

The aforementioned pill would instantly become a global bestseller. Unfortunately, exercise doesn't sell that well. The 2014 United States American National Health Interview Survey (NHIS) paints a dire picture. Among adults aged 18 and over, 30.2% of Americans are considered inactive with respect to aerobic activity guidelines and 19.8% of them are insufficiently active[ii].

Moreover, only 3.2% met full muscle-strengthening guidelines, 28.5% met full aerobic activity guidelines and just 21.4% met full guidelines for both aerobic activity and muscle strengthening.

According to a 2009 study[iii], the second most common barrier for exercise habit (after a lack of support) was a lack of willpower. Herein lies the difficulty in marketing exercise – something taking time and effort – when compared to a pill generating instant results.

Fortunately, while the magic pill doesn't exist, exercise does. It also isn't so hard to introduce into your life that you need to wait for the pill to appear. All you need are proven practical techniques and strategies to form a habit of exercise.

As the author of books like *How to Build Self-Discipline: Resist Temptations and Reach Your Long-Term Goals*, *Daily Self-Discipline: Everyday Habits and Exercises to Build Self-Discipline and Achieve Your Goals*, and *Self-Disciplined Dieter: How to Lose Weight and Become Healthy Despite Cravings and Weak Willpower*, self-discipline is my main area of expertise.

I want to help you break through the most common barriers for making exercise a part of your life and finally develop a permanent habit of it so you can become healthier, more vibrant, joyful, and enjoy other benefits regular physical exercise provides.

In the following pages you'll learn:

- how to get motivated to exercise. We'll dig deep into three different kinds of motivation, two additional opposing types of motivation, and how they can all help you get more active. We'll also cover practical strategies to handle procrastination;

- how to find time to exercise, which is a common reason why people are inactive. You'll learn about the horrible trade-off you're making when you don't exercise because of a lack of time. You'll also learn when to exercise and numerous non-obvious ways to make more time for exercise;

- how to stay motivated to exercise. Often it's easy to start, but hard to keep going. You'll learn a wide variety of ways to improve motivation, how to take a break and not destroy your habit of exercise, as well as discover how to prevent injuries, reduce soreness, and improve recovery so you can't make excuses because of pain;

- how to enjoy exercise. Tips on how to enjoy exercise are peppered throughout the book, but in this chapter we'll focus entirely on the simplest (and most effective) piece of advice that will most likely transform your entire attitude toward exercise (if you've always had trouble maintaining a regular exercise habit, it's possible you're the victim of this bad approach, often praised in fitness gyms);

- how to deal with other exercise-related issues like dealing with other people, managing your expectations related to physical activity, and dealing with discomfort, self-criticism, and feeling awkward when visiting the gym for the first time or trying a new sport.

If you haven't been exercising for a long time, chances are you've grown to believe exercise is not for you or that you're not strong enough – either mentally or physically – to act on the knowledge from this book.

Fortunately, nothing can be further from the truth, and there are simple – though not always easy – ways to fix this attitude. When put together and acted upon, the six chapters in this book – supported by over 80 references to scientific studies and credible experts – will help you form a new habit and make one of the most important changes you'll ever make in your life.

Let's embark on the journey now to learn how.

Chapter 1: How to Get Motivated to Exercise

If you're anything like most people struggling to get motivated to exercise, knowing that physical activity is good for you means nothing. You need something more to inspire you to get off the couch and move your body, but you're not sure what.

Out of all the challenges related to forming a habit of regular exercise, getting started is probably the most difficult thing. For this reason, this chapter will cover exactly how to overcome laziness or reluctance and start exercising.

We'll start with covering three different types of motivation and how they can help you start exercising. In addition to discussing them, we'll talk about push and pull motivations and how most people choose the wrong "P" and give up when they face obstacles.

Next, we'll dig deep into one of the most powerful ideas to get yourself motivated for exercise and keep exercising. With this simple – but slightly uncomfortable – trick you can light a fire under yourself that will ensure you'll get plenty of exercise.

Last but not least, we'll move on to the issue of procrastination and how to finally stop postponing exercise. It's tricky to start exercising if you have a habit of putting everything off for later. You'll learn how to make exercising an automated behavior so you don't have to exert your willpower each time you need to get active.

Without further ado, let's start by discussing three types of motivation: extrinsic, intrinsic, and prosocial.

Extrinsic Motivation

Extrinsic motivation is a common type of motivation, but doesn't usually work as well as people expect it to. It relates to motivation coming from the outcome you want to achieve[iv]. It's event-oriented, focused on the reward at the end of the road.

Competition is an example of extrinsic motivation. You don't compete for the sake of performing the activity (say, playing tennis), but to win the competition and receive a trophy.

Extrinsic motivation can be either about external rewards or punishments. In the most classic example, a student gets a good grade for performing well on a test and a bad grade when failing it.

When applied to exercise, reward-oriented extrinsic motivation can take the form of:

- your weight (a number on the scales can be surprisingly rewarding);

- waist circumference;

- status (bragging rights, inciting envy);

- drawing the attention of others (a person losing weight to attract a potential sexual partner);

- the "cool factor" (something – like yoga – is trendy and you want to be a part of it).

Punishment-oriented extrinsic motivation can take the form of:

- avoiding diseases related to obesity and/or a sedentary lifestyle;

- avoiding the pain of fat shaming;

- giving in to the pressure of a family member, friend, or colleague;

- losing a job opportunity;

- accountability (e.g. a $500 bet to lose x pounds).

For most people, extrinsic motivation is the primary source of motivation to start exercising. They either want to look good naked, avoid the pain of being "that" guy or gal, or because they want to impress others (say, at a high school reunion).

A good example of extrinsic motivation is accountability (discussed later). It can work wonders to introduce a regular habit of exercise when it's designed the right way.

Other ways to motivate yourself externally, like achieving status or avoiding diseases, are less effective. In the first case – doing something to gain status – the first obstacle will most likely make your motivation vanish. In the second case – avoiding diseases – it's usually too difficult to keep visualizing the potential risks of not exercising unless you've received a serious warning from your doctor. Unfortunately, extrinsic motivation only lasts as long as the reward is there or the threat of the punishment is real. The moment you achieve your ideal weight is usually the moment you lose motivation to keep exercising. After all, you've achieved your goal.

Moreover, research shows that extrinsic motivation is generally a poor source of inspiration.

A 2005 study on extrinsic and intrinsic motivators shows that extrinsic motivation led to poorer job performance than intrinsic motivation[v].

Another analysis in 2012 of over 200,000 U.S. public sector employees showed that using money as a motivator was less effective than using a passion or a challenge[vi]. In this analysis, intrinsic motivation was three times better than extrinsic motivation

Alternately, from the realm of weight loss, a 2012 study on financial incentives for weight loss has shown that small financial incentives for weight loss ($5.00 per percentage of initial weight lost) didn't increase motivation, while autonomous motivation (doing something out of your own will to better yourself) was consistently associated with greater weight losses[vii].

Does this mean that extrinsic motivation is useless? Not necessarily. It can't stand on its own legs, but it can be used in addition to intrinsic and/or prosocial motivation.

If you want to use extrinsic motivation to inspire yourself to keep going, it's better to focus on things that matter a lot to you. If you're obsessed with sports cars and you promised yourself you'll buy a new Porsche once you lose 30 pounds, this type of extrinsic motivation will be stronger than buying a new car just because you think you'll impress someone with it. Still, you should use this type of motivation as an additional motivator, not the only one.

Intrinsic Motivation

If extrinsic motivation is all about the external factors you can't control, intrinsic motivation is all about what's inside you. Namely, it deals with the desire to seek out new challenges, improve yourself, gain more knowledge, or assess your skills[viii].

Intrinsic motivation is long-lasting and most likely won't leave when you face insurmountable challenges. It's also self-sufficient, meaning there's nothing outside of yourself that affects it.

Some of the most common intrinsic motivators include:

- the desire to improve yourself (e.g. learn a new skill, feel stronger);

- enjoyment in the action (e.g. the rush from running or playing tennis);

- the challenge or assessment of your capabilities (e.g. doing a difficult climbing route);

- self-expression and creativity (e.g. sketching, creating music).

It's easy to come up with extrinsic motivators (looking better, making more money, achieving status), while intrinsic motivation is less tangible and more difficult to describe and quantify.

However, in the end, it's like the difference between feeling self-confident in an expensive car and feeling self-confident by believing in yourself. An expensive car can help you feel more confident, but it's an external factor that can be taken from you, consequently taking all of the perks like improved self-confidence with it.

If you want to maximize your chances of forming a regular habit of exercise, it's necessary to have at least one powerful intrinsic motivator.

The simplest way to find this motivator is to find a physical activity you love doing. Most people who struggle with getting exercise force themselves to go to the gym or attend fitness classes they hate. What they're doing is the total opposite of intrinsic motivation.

Introducing a habit of regular physical activity starts with finding activities you enjoy that you would practice even if they didn't give you any external rewards like better looks.

To further strengthen your intrinsic motivation, consider picking a physical activity that will teach you a new, challenging skill. It will combine your enjoyment of the activity with the desire to improve and challenge yourself, leading to a strong mix of intrinsic motivators.

For an example, my choice of sport is climbing. This kind of physical activity is not only fun (which is enough to fuel my motivation for regular exercise), but also forced me to learn a new way of moving my body, expressing my individual style through climbing. I constantly challenge myself by trying harder and harder routes.

It's both a physical and mental challenge that is perfect for long-lasting motivation. The additional benefits – improved physique and strength – are only a nice perk, not the end goals in themselves.

Now think of your regular 60-minute fitness class with exercises you hate and tell me if there's even a modicum of intrinsic motivation to find there. While climbing might not be your choice, try to find something that you can enjoy as much or more.

In 1997, researchers at the University of Rochester and the University of Southern Utah conducted a study on intrinsic motivation and exercise adherence[ix]. One group of participants participated in Tae Kwon Do classes while the other group attended classes of aerobics.

The first group adhered to their fitness routine better than the second one. It turned out they focused on enjoyment, competence, and social interaction –

all three being common intrinsic motivators for exercise.

As the scientists noted, "despite the fact that people primarily cite extrinsic reasons for exercising, intrinsic motivation remains a critical factor in sustained physical activity."

The implications of the study are clear and support the previously shared advice. In the scientists' words, "since session enjoyment predicts attendance and adherence, making exercise or physical activities more intrinsically motivating (i.e. fun, personally challenging) might be a viable route to enhancing persistence."

Prosocial Motivation

Prosocial motivation is the last kind of motivation and is usually left out when people discuss the types of motivation.

Professor Adam Grant, bestselling author of *Give and Take: A Revolutionary Approach to Success*[x], describes this type of motivation as "a desire to benefit other people and groups"[xi]. Neither extrinsic nor intrinsic motivation fully encompasses the idea of doing something out of a desire to help others, so prosocial motivation is a third kind of motivation.

Out of all the types of motivation, prosocial motivation is usually the strongest. Can you imagine somebody sacrificing herself to look good in the eyes of others or because she wants to express herself? How about a mother sacrificing her life for her children?

Prosocial motivation can take the form of:

- helping someone improve her circumstances (a husband taking care of his health so he can keep up with his active wife and participate in her favorite sports);

- helping someone avoid pain or suffering (a grandfather exercising to reduce the risk of a stroke so his grandchildren won't suffer because of his early death);

- doing something to support a certain cause (running a marathon to collect money to support a hospice).

While it's not necessary to have prosocial motivation to introduce a habit of regular exercise, prosocial motivation alone can be sufficient to stick to your habits forever.

A lifelong smoker can stop smoking overnight – without any other motivators – when his daughter tells him she wants him to be around – and not six feet deep – to walk her down the aisle.

Though it's for other people, please note this type of motivation is not about pressure – it's about your genuine desire to help somebody and not to avoid the pain of peer pressure. A husband trying to stop smoking because his wife nags at him every single day isn't benefiting from prosocial motivation. A husband who wants to stop smoking because he loves his wife and wants to be around her for a long time is.

When trying to introduce more physical activity in your life, consider who else could benefit from this change in your life. Keep this person in mind when tempted to give up or give in to laziness. It's a powerful motivator when you care about someone or something (a certain cause) to such an extent that it's more important in your eyes than you.

Push and Pull

Motivation can also be broken down into push motivation and pull motivation.

Push motivation is about pushing yourself to achieve a certain goal, while pull motivation is about being drawn to something you desire to such an extent that you can't help but keep working on your goals no matter what[xii].

In this sense, push motivation relies on your willpower – it's only as strong as your will to achieve the goal. In the case of pull motivation, willpower doesn't even come into play – you're so drawn to the thing you desire that you'll never stop until you achieve it.

It took me about six years of starting various businesses to develop a business sense and finally start a profitable company (and another, and another, and another). What motivated me wasn't the push – it was the pure pull, the desire to become a full-fledged, battle-tested entrepreneur. No matter the obstacles, problems, and other issues associated with the entrepreneur's roller coaster, I never considered dropping entrepreneurship – not even once.

How can you develop such a powerful pull motivation for exercise? That's the question I can't answer for you – it's something that's unique to your circumstances and personality. In my case, the allure of entrepreneurship has been pulling me ever since I was a kid. It is a clear example of a "pull" motivation.

Later on in my life, I've experienced the same thing when I was first introduced to indoor climbing. I didn't have to "push" myself to become better and go to the gym three to four times a week – the activity drew me in right away like an obsession.

What has always drawn you in fitness-wise, but you've never truly considered it in your life? Was it the beauty of Argentine tango? The smooth, controlled movements of a climber? The powerful mental battle of a marathoner and the subsequent unbeatable feeling of achievement?

Think of the things that draw you in and what kinds of physical activities can take you there. Don't push yourself to become a physically active person –

let the physical activity draw you in because of what it represents, what kind of a lifestyle it's associated with, or because of the concept behind it (like learning how to unleash your sexuality when dancing or looking inward when practicing yoga).

Please note that the push/pull distinction is slightly different than extrinsic and intrinsic motivation – it's not necessarily something you do because you enjoy it, but a goal that is so alluring that you can't help but do it.

Get Accountable from the Get Go

Accountability is one of the most powerful forms of extrinsic motivation. While intrinsic motivation will always get you farther and with fewer problems, strengthening it with accountability is an excellent idea to make self-change even easier, particularly if you've been living a sedentary lifestyle for a long time.

The easiest way to get accountable from the get go is to set financial stakes. There are sites that can help you stick to your resolutions such as www.stickK.com. You can also simply give a check or cash to your friend and let her spend it or send to a charity or an organization you don't support (so there's an even better incentive not to fail) if you don't keep your word.

Be specific about what you want to achieve and the deadline. The idea only works if there's no way to renegotiate the contract – you either achieve the goal or lose the money. The pain of losing it once will strengthen your resolve the next time you're tempted to give up again.

Another way to become accountable from the start is to start exercising with a friend.

A study conducted by Brandon C. Irwin at the Michigan State University and his colleagues has shown that exercising with a partner improves performance on aerobic exercises due to the Köhler effect, a phenomenon that occurs when a person works harder as a member of a group than when working alone[xiii].

However, when you choose to exercise with a partner who's similar to you in terms of physical activity, there's a risk you'll allow each other excuses not to go and exercise.

For this reason, find a more demanding fitness pal, ideally someone with an already developed fitness routine that will push you to exercise. A 2012 study suggests that working out with a slightly better partner makes individuals more persistent[xiv], so for best results, find someone slightly more athletic to help you stick to your new habit.

How to Deal With and Overcome Procrastination

Putting off physical activity is typical among people who don't have a regular habit of exercise.

There are three common reasons for procrastination:

1. You're not looking forward to the exercise because you dislike it.

Out of the three most common reasons for putting exercise off, this one is the easiest to solve. Just like some people find dozens of other tasks when they're supposed to study for a boring exam, so some people find something else to do when they're supposed to exercise.

It's a great example of a lack of intrinsic motivation (not getting pure enjoyment out of exercise). If you've recently started practicing a new sport but you're rarely motivated to go out and practice it, chances are it's not the right kind of physical activity for you.

The right type of exercise should draw you in and ideally, make you obsessed about it from the get go. If you're performing it in the afternoon or the evening, it shouldn't be something that hangs over your head as yet another thing on the to-do list. It should be something you're looking forward to and would like to happen sooner.

In a sense, procrastination can be a useful tool to help you determine what works for you and what doesn't. If you always procrastinate before studying, perhaps you're studying the wrong things. If you always procrastinate on writing essays and replace it with, say, programming, perhaps it's your subconscious telling you that your strength lies in programming and writing essays is a distraction.

You won't solve the problem of procrastination if you don't find the type of exercise that feels *right*. As mentioned before, the idea of enjoying exercise is one of the most important concepts to introduce a regular habit of physical activity. We'll be talking about it in greater detail in a later chapter. That's where you'll learn how to beat procrastination if it's because of this reason.

2. Exercise is not automatic to you.

Even if you know that exercise is good for you and that you'll feel great during and after it, you may still procrastinate.

The reason for this behavior is usually that it's not an automated behavior for you, and consequently you need willpower to get started. Since the level of your willpower varies, it's easy to procrastinate even when it comes to the exercises you like.

The underlying problem here is not the activity in itself, but getting yourself prepared to do it – putting on your fitness gear, driving to your local climbing gym, or loading your playlist for a jogging session.

The solution is simple – you need to make exercise so automatic it feels like brushing your teeth or taking a shower during your morning routine. No matter your willpower levels, you don't struggle with these things because they're a part of your automated routine, right?

According to Charles Duhigg, the author of *The Power of Habit: Why We Do What We Do in Life and Business*[xv], a habit consists of three elements: cue (trigger), action, and reward.

James Clear, a writer and researcher on behavioral psychology, habit formation, and performance improvement, calls it the 3 R's of habit formation – reminder (cue or trigger), routine (action), and reward[xvi].

In the case of exercise, the cue would be seeing your running shoes by the bed in the morning, the action would be putting them on and going out for a jog, and the reward would be the rush of endorphins. When set up properly, it's a self-reinforcing mechanism that makes the habit more and more automated until it becomes as natural as brushing your teeth in the morning.

It takes consistent practice to develop a habit, but once it's a part of your daily routine, you'll no longer suffer from procrastination-related problems. Pick a cue that will always be the same and that you'll always follow with a specific action that will be reinforced with a specific reward.

Some good cues to consider:

- a specific time on a specific day. For example, I go swimming either on Tuesday or Thursday at 7 in the morning. After following such a routine for several weeks or months, you can't help but do it out of habit.

- a reminder on your phone (ideally with a distinct sound or a song). I used to play a specific song and do push-ups while listening to it. To this day, the song still reminds me of push-ups.

- an existing behavior. For instance, if you meditate in the morning, it can serve as a cue to exercise right after finishing your session.

When starting out with a new habit of exercise, start small. You don't have to start by introducing a habit of running for 60 minutes every single day. Even running five minutes around the neighborhood is enough to make a new behavior automatic. In fact, it's better to start as small as possible so there's very little (if any) resistance to it. As Leo Babauta, blogger at ZenHabits.net puts it, "make it so easy you can't say no"[xvii].

What's important is not the action in itself, but building the self-reinforcing habit. If you already have a habit of exercising one minute a day, it will be much easier to turn it into 2, 5 or 10 minutes than starting a new habit of exercising for 10 minutes right away.

Lastly, don't forget about a proper reward. An unhealthy snack after exercise is not a good idea since it won't help you reach your ultimate goal of improving your health.

Thankfully, if you choose the right type of exercise for you, the feeling of enjoyment will be the only reward you'll ever need. Alternatively, reward yourself with a healthy meal, a nap, massage, an evening out with friends – anything that makes you feel good while not ruining your fitness progress.

3. You're used to a sedentary lifestyle.

If you've been living a sedentary lifestyle for a large portion of your life, don't expect to become a fitness machine in a week. Start as small as possible and work on eliminating resistance to exercise.

Simple choices to move a little bit more during the day (taking the stairs instead of the elevator, not driving if you can walk there in 5 to 10 minutes) can reactivate your willingness to become more active. Don't schedule these "exercises." Just replace your existing behaviors with less convenient, but still manageable changes to introduce more physical activity in your life.

Don't expect to feel no resistance to exercise if it's been months or years since you've last engaged in physical activity, just as you shouldn't expect to pull yourself up 10 times if you've never done a pull-up in your life.

Start slowly and let the resistance melt by a tiny amount each day until you no longer find it challenging to introduce a deliberate habit of exercise. If you rush things, you'll only increase the risk of an injury or soreness and a subsequent bad association with exercise.

HOW TO GET MOTIVATED TO EXERCISE: QUICK RECAP

1. Extrinsic motivation is focused on rewards and punishments. It can take the form of achieving a specific weight or waist circumference, attracting a sexual partner, avoiding diseases, avoiding pressure from others, or even a financial bet.

For most people, extrinsic motivation is not sufficient to help introduce a regular habit of exercising. It can be a worthy addition to a set of strong intrinsic and/or prosocial motivators, though.

2. Intrinsic motivation is focused on what's inside you. In this sense, it's self-sufficient since nothing controls it but you. Intrinsic motivation can take the form of the desire to improve, enjoy, or challenge yourself. It can also be for self-analysis or self-expression.

Intrinsic motivation is the primary fuel you can use to introduce a habit of exercise. Start with picking an activity that you genuinely enjoy and that you would do even if it wasn't associated with other rewards like better looks, more status, etc.

3. Prosocial motivation is focused on the desire to help others. You want to do something so you can better someone else's life, help someone else avoid pain, or support a cause you believe in. It's usually the strongest and most long-lasting source of motivation that will fuel you no matter the circumstances.

To find your own prosocial motivators, think of people close to you who would benefit from your change (for example, your kids will get to enjoy more physical activity with you as a companion, and consequently grow up to be healthy, active adults). Think of your "why" person each time you're tempted to give up. If it's no longer about you, but primarily somebody else, it's easier to stick to your new resolutions.

4. You can push yourself toward a specific goal or let it pull you. Push motivation is usually weaker because it depends on your willpower, and the moment it runs out, your motivation is gone, too. Pull motivation is better because instead of exerting your

willpower to reach a goal, you let the goal draw you in.

In exercise, you can benefit from pull motivation by discovering a type of a physical activity that represents something that lures you in. It can be a certain process, the concept behind it, or a lifestyle associated with it.

5. Accountability is an example of a very effective type of extrinsic motivation. While it's not entirely necessary to help you achieve your goals, it's a valuable addition for people with a weak resolve. Two types of accountability you can introduce in your life are setting financial stakes and having a fitness partner.

In the first case, the fear of losing money will prevent you from giving up. In the second case, your partner (ideally someone better than you) will be your drill sergeant, pushing you to keep going and holding you accountable.

6. Procrastination is usually caused by choosing the wrong type of an exercise, not having an automated behavior, or being so used to laziness that

all attempts at change cause overwhelming resistance. To solve these problems, make sure you look forward to your exercise, develop a habit, and gradually reduce resistance by introducing tiny changes in your daily routine.

Chapter 2: How to Find Time to Exercise

You'd love to start exercising, but you can't find enough time to do it. In fact, you're having a hard time completing other important tasks, let alone adding yet another regular activity to your schedule.

If only you had more time, you could introduce more physical activity in your life. But is it really the underlying issue here or are there some ways in which you can find some time to exercise regularly? That's what we'll cover in this chapter.

We'll start with an extremely important idea that should stay at the forefront of your mind each time you say "I don't have time to exercise."

We'll discuss the most optimal times of the day for exercise and discuss the difference between quick exercises and time-consuming ones (and how to adjust them to fit in your busy schedule).

Lastly, I'll give you some specific tips on how you can make more time for exercise – even if you're extremely busy and can't spare even 15 minutes a day.

The First Step: Prioritizing Health

Exercise can be time-consuming, and for busy people, it may be extremely challenging to introduce even 15 minutes of exercise a day. However, that's looking at things from the short-term perspective.

Whenever you say you don't have time to exercise, you're expressing that you value your health less than whatever else keeps you busy. However, when asked about your values you wouldn't say that work is your number one priority, would you? Most people put health at the top of their core life values. Yet, their daily routines don't reflect it.

As the saying goes, if you don't make time for health, you'll have to make time for illness. It's 100% true. Numerous studies show that a lack of exercise is a major cause of sickness.

For instance, a 2012 paper says that "the body rapidly maladapts to insufficient physical activity, and if continued, results in substantial decreases in both total and quality years of life. Taken together, conclusive evidence exists that physical inactivity is one important cause of most chronic diseases. In addition, physical activity primarily prevents, or delays, chronic diseases, implying that chronic disease need not be an inevitable outcome during life"[xviii].

Another 2012 article on the effects of physical inactivity on major non-communicable diseases worldwide has estimated that physical inactivity causes 6% of the burden of disease from coronary heart disease, 7% of type 2 diabetes, 10% of breast cancer, and 10% of colon cancer. In general, inactivity causes 9% of premature mortality[xix].

These numbers are very conservative as the data regarding levels of physical activity was self-reported, and people notoriously overestimate how much exercise they get the same way people underreport how much they eat.

A 2015 study of over 334,000 European men and women has found that twice as many deaths may be attributable to lack of physical activity than to the number of obesity-related deaths[xx]. The authors of the study shared a surprising fact that doing exercise equivalent to a 20-minute brisk walk each day (burning between 90 and 110 calories) would take a physically inactive person to a "moderately inactive" group, which would reduce her risk of premature death by 16 to 30%.

I could cite scientific research about the dangers of physical inactivity all day long, but I think I've already proven my point – you can't afford *not* to exercise, and a lack of time is no reason for not doing it.

Let's say you save two and a half hours a week (the Department of Health and Human Services' recommended amount of weekly physical activity[xxi]) by not exercising. That's about 22 minutes a day, or 130 hours a year.

Sounds like a lot?

Then consider how much time it would take you to recover if you became ill due to a lack of physical activity. Even a simple cold can result in a few days of decreased productivity and additional money spent on medication. And we're not even talking about chronic diseases that cost thousands a year and hundreds of hours wasted on doctor visits, regular check-ups, time spent researching how to make yourself feel better, etc.

If you put these calculations in your mind and remind yourself of them each time you say "I don't have time for exercise," you'll realize you're making a bad trade between saving 22 minutes a day and potentially losing more time later on because you're feeling horrible.

In addition, we still haven't even considered additional bad sides of physical inactivity such as:

- a weaker ability to deal with stress, anxiety, and/or depression (exercise can alleviate symptoms among clinically depressed[xxii], reduce anxiety sensitivity[xxiii] and treat depression and anxiety[xxiv])

- lowered perception of your attractiveness (exercise improves self-worth in women[xxv], and is even more effective when done outdoors[xxvi])

- weaker brainpower (exercise improves cognitive function in young adult males[xxvii] and prevents cognitive decline that begins after age 45[xxviii])

-   lower productivity (exercise increases productivity[xxix] and energy[xxx])

-   worse creativity (exercise enhances creativity[xxxi])

- worse sleep (exercise improves sleep[xxxii])

Yet you'd rather save 22 minutes a day than tremendously improve the quality of your life and help you do more in less time? Besides, this list is only a small selection of all the benefits provided by physical activity.

If I told you that investing 25 minutes a day in exercise would give you an additional hour of productivity each day, would you still lack time for exercise? If I sold you 60 dollars for 25 dollars, would you tell me you don't have the money?

When Should You Work Out?

Most people who have regular working hours choose to exercise either in the morning or in the late afternoon or evening. There are benefits and drawbacks to each of these periods, so consider the advice I'll share below as a general guideline to adapt to your daily schedule.

Working out in the morning

Benefits:

The primary benefit of working out in the morning is that you have plenty of energy. It's more tempting to forgo exercise in the afternoon or in the evening when you're tired after an entire day of working or taking care of chores.

Moreover, if you work out in the morning, you're done with the exercise for the day – it's out of your head and you no longer have to remember to do it.

It also doesn't hinder your social life (not many want to meet at seven in the morning) and gives you something to be proud of right after waking up, giving you a nice feeling of being productive.

In the case of working out at the local gym, an additional benefit is that it's empty or has very few people. The vision of a crowded gym in late afternoon doesn't motivate, does it.

Physical activity in the morning – on an empty stomach – is also beneficial for weight loss. As a

2013 British study has shown, people can burn up to 20% more body fat by exercising in the morning on an empty stomach[xxxiii].

Drawbacks:

Time in the morning is usually limited, and if you want to practice a sport that can only be done at a specific venue (say, climb in a climbing gym) it's possible it won't be open yet. For this reason, mornings are better for exercise that doesn't take a lot of time and can be either done at home, in the area, or in a place that's open very early (like a fitness gym).

In some cases, morning workouts can also pose a bigger challenge to your willpower than the afternoon. It can be dreadful to wake up early in the morning, realize it's below freezing outside, and leave your warm bed to exercise.

Lastly, mornings are not friendly for team sports. These are usually done in the late afternoon or in the evening, and you shouldn't expect to convince your entire team to have a match at six in the morning.

Suggestions:

Physical activities that work well in the morning include:

- jogging or brisk walking (including Nordic walking). You don't need to do it in a specific place (though obviously doing it in a forest or a park is more pleasant than running through the city) and it's a nice way to begin your day. Even a 20-30 minute session is enough to get you energized for the day ahead and takes care of your body's needs for physical activity for a given day;

- any type of exercise done at home, with either machines or free weights. If you have a stationary bike, cycling for 20-30 minutes can jumpstart your day. If you have a home gym (or a gym in your garage or basement), then it should be your first choice for exercise in the morning. An effective weightlifting session shouldn't last longer than 45 minutes, and it's perfect to give your body a proper dose of exercise;

- yoga, pilates, tai chi, and similar types of exercise are also perfect to perform in the morning. They are not only a good way to get your body moving, but also enter a quasi-meditative state that will calm you down and prepare for the day ahead;

- biking. A quick bike ride in the morning before heavy traffic hits the streets (if there's no park or wilderness area close to you) can be an invigorating and relaxing experience;

- stretching exercises (including foam rolling). If you don't have a lot of time, at least try to do a few basic stretches. I usually do foam rolling in the morning to reduce the tension in my muscles (I spend more time talking about foam rolling in my book *How to Relax*);

- swimming. Many swimming pools open early in the morning. If you suffer from back pain – like many people nowadays do – you should swim regularly. A 1996 Japanese study on swimming and back pain showed that more than 90% of the patients felt they had improved after 6 months participation in a swimming program[xxxiv]. A 2009 Finnish systematic review has also confirmed that swimming can be potentially beneficial to patients suffering from chronic low back pain as well as pregnancy-related low back pain[xxxv].

These are just a few suggestions, and there are many more sports that can work in the morning. For instance, if you play tennis and there's a tennis backboard near you (or if you have a partner who also wakes up early), it can be an enjoyable morning routine to get your blood pumping and improve your skills.

Moreover, if you don't have to go to work in the morning, you have many more options to choose from – especially if you have a fitness pal, a friend, or a spouse who also doesn't have to go to work in the morning.

Working out in the afternoon or in the evening
Benefits:

The biggest benefit of working out in the afternoon is that as long as you've taken care of other things planned for the day, you're free to practice a certain sport without strict time limits. It enables you to engage in more time-consuming sports, team sports, or physical activities of a more social nature.

While technically you can go bouldering in the morning (if your gym is open early enough), a large part of the enjoyment from this sport comes from the fact you're doing it with other people.

The same applies to other sports that you usually do with other people like all kinds of extreme sports (skateboarding, surfing, kitesurfing, etc.), all team sports (you can practice most of them alone, but not play them), martial arts, golf, and other social kinds of physical activity like dancing.

Drawbacks:

The biggest drawback of physical activity in the afternoon or in the evening is that people usually have less energy after 5 PM, especially after 8 hours of work.

If you can't exercise in the morning, and afternoon or evening are your only options, make sure that the sport you're going to practice is something you look forward to. A good test of whether a certain activity is for you is whether you think about it during the day – do you look forward to it or dread it?

In the past, I was forced to practice judo in the evening as a part of my curriculum at the college. I dreaded each day because I didn't enjoy it. I consider myself a self-disciplined person (I wouldn't write books about self-discipline otherwise, right?), but even for me it's challenging to exercise in the afternoon or evening if it's something I don't enjoy.

Another drawback of exercising later in the day is that many venues where you practice sports are crowded in the afternoon or evening. This can result in a frustrating experience that will discourage you from exercise.

Swimming is a regular part of my weekly schedule, but I never do it in the afternoon because I don't look forward to swimming in a crowded swimming pool. It's much calmer in the early morning when I can have the entire lane for myself.

When thinking about what kinds of sports to practice in the afternoon or the evening, don't forget about this aspect. Sometimes it's better to wait until the late evening to perform your workout than go in the afternoon, get angry at the crowds, and have a less than optimal workout, which is a common thing at a fitness gym during peak hours.

Suggestions:

Most of the sports I recommended performing in the morning can also be done in the afternoon or in the evening, especially if you go after more volume (a solid 90-minute long bike ride in the afternoon compared to a brief 20-minute bike ride in the morning).

However, if you have a more relaxed afternoon or evening, you can spend this time practicing a more involved sport for longer than just 20-30 minutes so you can get a bigger dose of exercise in one session.

Having the best of both worlds

If your days tend to get busy in the afternoon, morning exercise (at least 20-30 minutes) should be a must-have part of your daily routine with afternoon exercise an additional option to squeeze in more exercise time if you can afford it.

If you exercise 20 minutes each day in the morning and add one 2-hour session on a more relaxed Friday or two 1-hour sessions on Saturday and Sunday, you'll get enough exercise in any given week to enjoy its numerous benefits.

I'm a huge fan of having specific days designated to certain sports. If you can do it, pick specific days during the week (and ideally specific hours) to practice specific sports. Schedule them in your calendar and don't let anything interfere with your plans. Understand that it's not about being selfish – it's precisely the total opposite of it. By exercising, you become a better person so you can better serve others.

I go to the gym every Monday, Wednesday, and Friday morning. My routine never changes. Years of following such a routine have made going to the gym not just an option – it's something I have to do or I'll feel there's something missing. If you also set specific days for exercise and faithfully exercise on them, within a few months you'll experience the same thing.

If there's no way you can find time to exercise during the weekday, schedule exercise for your weekends. Saturdays and Sundays are perfect for practicing physical activities that aren't necessarily sports. For instance, consider a day trip to a nearby wild area.

Hiking is a non-sport physical activity that can be very demanding but extremely gratifying and provide a powerful bonding experience when done with family or friends.

Even if you can't afford practicing any kind of a sport regularly for various reasons, hiking or even taking 1-hour long walks on Saturdays and Sundays should be possible, and still take you from an inactive person to a person getting at least the minimum recommended amount of physical activity.

Quick Exercises vs Time-Consuming Sports

There are countless workout plans for busy people: 7-minute workouts, 5-minute workouts, 3-minute workouts, and so on. While these plans do serve a purpose if you follow them, consider these quick exercises a way to make sure you'll get *some* exercise during the day, not *all of it*.

A sport or other physical activity you practice regularly and can do for hours without looking at the clock is what will help you develop a permanent habit of exercise. Quick exercises rarely (if ever) produce a feeling of excitement. Have you ever looked forward to a session of leg lunges or jumping jacks?

20 minutes of bodyweight exercises in the morning each day is great. It's enough to start your day on the right note and feel productive. However, adding even just one or two 60- to 90-minute sessions of exercises you enjoy more (for instance, swimming or playing tennis or cycling) is what takes you from one, less healthy category to another, healthier one (say, mildly active to moderately active).

For this reason, I highly recommend not settling with a generic workout plan just so you can maintain your fitness levels. Find something that will fire you up and not only make you maintain your current physical activity, but inspire you to surpass your fitness goals.

How to Make More Time for Exercise

If you're struggling with a lack of time, below are some of the most effective tips you can use to make more time for exercise. It's not a question of finding more time because we all get the same amount of hours in the day – it's about using your time more wisely, and that's what the advice below is about.

Delegate regular tasks

There are certain chores you either do daily or weekly that take up a lot of time you could otherwise spend exercising. While hiring someone to perform all of them would probably be too expensive for many people, hiring someone to spend two or three hours a week to clean your home shouldn't pose a problem for the monthly budget.

Consider it an investment in your health. If you can free up two or three hours a week that you can spend exercising, you'll reduce the risk of numerous preventable, costly diseases. Weekly cleaning costs nothing when compared to high medical-related costs (including insurance, doctor visits, prescriptions, lost time, etc.).

You can find help with services like the TaskRabbit app or on sites with classifieds. Alternatively, look for a local maid services company.

This piece of advice is even more important for entrepreneurs and freelancers who work at home and spend time doing low-output tasks that could be outsourced to others, thus enabling you to spend more time on high-output activities.

If you're having a hard time outsourcing some of your daily or weekly tasks, calculate your hourly rate and consider how much cleaning costs you a week in terms of lost income. If you're not willing to work for less than $50 per hour, but you spend 2 hours a week cleaning (that would cost $50 when hiring a home cleaner), you're losing $50 a week.

Replace daily habits

Let's assume there's absolutely no way you can make time for exercise with your current schedule. You have so many things to do, and it's impossible to get rid of any of these tasks. Okay, fine. Then how about replacing how you perform certain daily habits?

There's the age old idea of bike commuting. I'm not a huge proponent of it (just because I understand how bike-unfriendly some cities can be and how horrible it is to cycle during the winter), but it can be an option to consider during the spring and summer. Often, you can get to work more quickly on your bike than in your car because you can skip the heavy traffic.

One of the tennis courts I go to is about 20 minutes away from my apartment by car. When I once rode a bike there during peak hours, it took me maybe five minutes more and I got an additional 50 minutes of exercise while spending just 10 minutes more on it when compared to driving.

Another idea is that when you need to have a long phone call, go on a walk. You're going to spend this time on the phone anyway, so why not take a walk if you don't need to have anything specific (documents, computer, etc.) within your reach?

Create a home gym or reduce the number of trips home

If you don't have time to go to the gym, create a gym in your home, garage, or basement. I have a gym in my basement. If I didn't have it, I would have to spend an additional 30 minutes driving to a local gym, which would add up to 90 minutes a week of wasted time.

Buying basic equipment will probably be more expensive than a monthly pass to the gym, but you'll quickly recoup your investment by saving time and money on future gym passes. It's also easier on your willpower if you have a gym in a room nearby and not in a building a few miles away.

If you can't set up a home gym, carry your gym gear (or anything else you need to practice the sport of your choice) in your car so you don't need another trip home after work.

My friend often has an Aerobie (a flying ring) in the trunk of his car during the summer. If we meet up, we can take it and throw it to each other, thus getting some enjoyable exercise while catching up.

Have active dates and meet-ups

Who said that you always have to meet with your friends for coffee or go on a date to a restaurant? Get more creative. Take your date or your friend somewhere else where you both can get some exercise and enjoy yourselves. Consider:

- a hiking trip with a friend. Best left for the weekends, it's a great way to get some exercise and recharge your batteries.

- indoor climbing with a date. Stand out by taking him or her to a more exciting place than a local restaurant or cinema.

- weekend kayaking with your partner. Explore the world from a different perspective and get some adrenaline pumping.

- buy an Aerobie, a Frisbee on steroids. It's a fun way to spend a weekend afternoon with a group, friends, or your family.

- take a walk. If you're going to meet with your friend and talk anyway, why not talk while walking around the local lake, in a park, or on a forest trail?

- go cycling. That's one of the primary ways I get exercise during the spring and summer with one of my friends. During the colder months, we replace it with walks.

Get a pedometer

Most new smartphones can be turned into a pedometer with a free app. Once you're aware of the number of steps you take every single day, you can turn it into a game – while not necessarily spending a lot more time on it (for instance, you'll choose stairs over the elevator so you can clock in more steps).

A rule of a thumb is to get 10,000 steps a day. Remember that you not only take steps when exercising, but also when doing your daily chores or just walking about the house.

If you're into numbers and data, consider buying a proper fitness tracker. The more you can gamify exercise, the easier it will be to start and keep doing it – while not necessarily spending more time during the day on it.

Do exercise in micro amounts

If you're extremely busy, you can still squeeze in a few minutes of exercise a day. For instance, install a pull-up bar in your home and do a pull-up (or just do the negative phase of the movement by lowering your body) each time you pass it. It will add up to at least a few reps a day, and that's at least *some* exercise you wouldn't otherwise get.

Another idea is to take micro breaks (1-2 minutes) every 30-60 minutes or so to do 10 squats or a few push-ups or just walk around the office or your home.

Again, this type of exercise shouldn't become your primary way of getting some physical activity, but it's still valuable if you can't afford spending more time on exercise on a given day.

HOW TO FIND TIME TO EXERCISE: QUICK RECAP

1. Exercise provides a plethora of health benefits and protects from a multitude of diseases and health disorders. Spending even just 25 minutes a day on exercise (the minimum recommended amount of physical activity) will increase your productivity and protect you from dozens of hours wasted on being sick or feeling suboptimal.

Physical activity is not the question of whether you have time, but whether you can recognize the value of this investment. Thanks to improved energy, focus, creativity, and mood, 25 minutes a day can result in an additional hour (if not more) of productive time.

2. Working out in the morning should become a part of your daily routine – even if it's just 15 minutes of stretching or a 20-minute bike ride. People who are always busy run the risk of not being able to squeeze in exercise time in the afternoons or evenings. It's easier to wake up 20 minutes earlier and do your

exercises than exert willpower or shift your schedule to exercise at the end of the day.

3. While mornings are best for quick exercises you may not necessarily look forward to, afternoon and evening workouts should be all about things that are fun.

If you're looking forward to your session at the end of the day, you won't need to use your willpower to exercise. Not only that – you'll actually consider it something that recharges you, something that you can't wait to happen. That drive will quickly make it a permanent, unbreakable habit.

4. Don't forget about the weekends. If there's absolutely no way you can find time to exercise during the week, you have no excuses to find one to two hours each Saturday and Sunday to exercise. It doesn't have to be a specific sport – even a simple long walk or going for a hike will help get your body moving and deliver the health benefits associated with physical activity.

5. You can use your time more wisely to make more time for exercise. The primary ways to do so

include delegating certain tasks (like cleaning), replacing daily habits (doing the same things, but in a more active way such as choosing your bike over your car), setting up a home gym or carrying fitness gear with you, having active dates and meet-ups with friends (instead of just going to a local café), using a pedometer that will turn daily activities into a fun game, and doing exercises in micro amounts such as 5 push-ups each hour.

Chapter 3: How to Stay Motivated to Exercise

You've started exercising or have been exercising for some time already, but you could use some help to keep your motivation.

In this chapter you'll learn how to make exercise a part of your lifestyle and keep looking forward to it even after months or years after introducing this habit in your life.

While ups and downs happen with each habit, you too can establish a reliable, lifelong habit that will never again go away – just like brushing your teeth or combing your hair.

Set Goals

Whether you've been working out for a few weeks, a few months, or a few years, a set of goals is always a useful thing to have.

Your goals should be SMART (Specific, Measurable, Achievable, Realistic, and Time-bound). For instance, if you're new to jogging, your goal can be to run a mile without breaking a sweat by the third month of your workouts.

If you've just started swimming, set a goal to swim 10 laps in a row by your tenth session. If you're climbing, your goal can be to finish five more difficult routes at the gym by the end of the next month. If you started playing tennis, it can be serving three balls correctly in a row.

These goals are simple ways to introduce structure and a system of tracking your efforts so you can actually see your progress, which is one of the most important things that will motivate you to keep going.

Your goals don't necessarily have to be related to the sport itself. They can also be related to your appearance (have a flat stomach by the end of the year) or a general sense of well-being (no more feeling tired the entire day after six months of consecutive workouts).

When I started swimming regularly for the first time in my life (before, I usually went to a swimming pool once every few weeks or months, so I wasn't a good swimmer), I set a goal to swim 5 laps in a row using one style, then 5 laps using another. On my next workout, I increased it to 6 laps. I slowly kept adding more laps until I could swim for an entire hour without stopping.

The feeling of accomplishment helped me stick to swimming during the most difficult early period of exercise when it was hard to spend an entire hour swimming with no breaks.

Easy goal setting and the ability to see quick progress is what makes certain sports more exciting than others. In indoor climbing, the sheer amount of different routes and completely different skills needed to master them is what fires you up to keep training.

I recently finished a route I was trying to complete during almost every single session in the last three weeks. The feeling of exhilaration upon completing it made me even more addicted to climbing and motivated me to set new goals with harder and harder routes.

If you're new to a specific sport, learn what goals are achievable within a relatively short time frame (say, a month or so), and focus on achieving them. Fast progress when you're a beginner is immensely helpful when trying to develop a habit of regular physical activity.

Keep It Fresh and Challenging

If you've been practicing a given sport for a long period of time, things can get stale.

Some sports are easier to keep fresh than others. In climbing, there's always a new environment to test your skills, new routes to master, holds or footholds that require more practice. It can take years before you first experience burnout.

In some activities, you might need more creativity to come up with ways to make your workouts fun and challenging again. In addition to setting "regular" long-term goals, add objectives that can quickly lead to visible improvements.

In tennis, you can set a goal to improve your forehand, but if it's already great, then the improvements will probably be too small to notice quickly (and thus, not very motivating). While practicing your forehand to make it even better should remain a part of your routine, setting an additional goal related to a different skill – for instance, smashes – will inject a bit more fun into your sessions.

In jogging, consider switching regular jogging with sprints or hill sprints. Completely change your route. Start jogging with someone else. Change your playlist (or switch from music to podcasts). Work on improving your speed and not just endurance.

In cycling, make sure to vary your routes – ride uphill, downhill, longer routes, shorter ones, and so on. If you constantly go on the same exact bike ride, things are guaranteed to get boring quickly.

When practicing your chosen sport, switch your focus to something fresh to introduce newness in your workouts.

For instance, when I go climbing, I not only try completely different routes requiring skills I use rarely, but also sometimes give myself a specific "theme" for the day – for instance, balancing or footwork. With just a few such themes (footwork day, balance day, finger day, overhanging walls day, or endurance day with more traversing), it's easy to make each of your workouts distinct and more interesting.

Don't forget about the "challenging" part. When you're a beginner, everything is challenging, so everything is motivating. Your first proper serve in tennis, your first scaled wall, your first mile of jogging, it's all new.

Yet, when you already have some skills, there's temptation to stick to what's easy and no longer have what the Zen Buddhists call the "beginner's mind" or *shoshin*. Zen teacher Shunryu Suzuki writes in his book *Zen Mind, Beginner's Mind*, "In the beginner's mind there are many possibilities, in the expert's mind there are few"[xxxvi].

Practice with an open mind and readiness to get the most out of new opportunities for improvement. An attitude of eagerness and openness will keep boredom out of your workouts while guaranteeing further growth and fun.

Get the Chain Going

An unknown touring comic realized that to get better at his vocation, he had to write new jokes on a daily basis. He formed his habit by putting a big red X in his calendar each day he succeeded writing a new joke.

After several days, he noticed a short chain of X's forming in his calendar. As silly as it sounds, he didn't want his chain to break, so he kept writing new jokes and crossing off days in his calendar. A few weeks later his new routine was established.

Today, Jerry Seinfeld is one of the most famous American comics. His technique[xxxvii] can help you stay motivated to exercise, too.

Skipping one day makes it easier to skip the next. Then the next, and the next, and your habit is gone. Try Seinfeld's technique and set a goal to develop a long chain in your calendar (search for "don't break the chain" or "chain calendar" or "habit streak" for useful apps for your phone if you don't use a physical calendar).

Sometimes simple reminders are enough to keep going, and you only have to keep going for several months at most to build a permanent habit that won't go away the moment you skip it for one day.

Have an Alternative for Lazy Days

Lazy days, when you're not in the mood to work out, can happen – particularly in the first few months of establishing your new habits.

If you don't feel like going to the gym, putting on your running shoes, or packing your swimming gear, have an alternative, low-resistance type of exercise you can do in place of your primary activity.

Many people have the "all or nothing" mentality with exercise. However, it's not about one event, but about the process. Some exercise is better than none.

If you can't make yourself go to the gym, some bodyweight exercises at home are still better than doing nothing altogether. They keep your chain going and support the process of establishing your new habit.

If you skip your workout entirely and don't do any other kind of exercise, you can create a precedent, thus making it easier to not exercise the next time you feel lazy.

Life isn't always smooth sailing. On some days – even if you usually look forward to your session of exercise – you won't feel like doing it. Breaking through the resistance and doing it anyway is what enforces your habit and makes you tougher.

As Rocky Balboa says in *Rocky Balboa*, "You, me, or nobody is gonna hit as hard as life. But it ain't about how hard you hit. It's about how hard you can get hit and keep moving forward. How much you can take and keep moving forward. That's how winning is done."

In an ideal world, you'd always break through the resistance. In the real world, if you can't gather enough strength to act despite laziness, it's better to do something than nothing.

You can replace going to the gym with a few bodyweight exercises at home. You can swim for 15 minutes in a lake nearby instead of going for a full hour to the swimming pool. You can have a quick 20-minute jog around the block instead of your usual 90-minute route, or even just do a few leg exercises at home (say, with a jump rope).

This piece of advice also applies to general days where you feel you're lacking strength or energy –

not necessarily because of laziness. Exercising at 75%, 50%, or 25% intensity or volume is still better than not doing it at all.

Sometimes when I go swimming, I don't feel my energy is at 100%. Instead of leaving the pool and going home, I either just do fewer laps and take longer breaks, switch to a less demanding swimming style for a few laps, or try something else (e.g. diving).

Don't fall victim to the "all or nothing" mentality. It's fine to do something easier on the days you don't feel like doing anything at all. Just make an effort to do *something*.

Keep Records

A 2011 paper on weight loss and engagement with a web-based food and exercise diary has shown that people who used the self-monitoring tools often were more likely to achieve weight loss than those who didn't use them as frequently[xxxviii].

I keep a workout log for my weightlifting sessions and note down the weights lifted each session. It makes it easy to track my progress, and it feels good to see small improvements in each training cycle.

I use a simple Excel spreadsheet for my own workout log, but there's a huge selection of apps you can download on your phone to keep records of your workouts.

The most popular fitness apps for joggers or people who walk a lot not only work as a pedometer, but also keep the details of each session like distance traveled, speed, calories burned, and so on.

Other apps make it easy to track and increase weights lifted during each session for optimum intensity or simply keep you more accountable by letting you cross off each day with a workout.

Reward Yourself

Small rewards at the end of each workout can increase your motivation on the days you don't feel like working out.

Sometimes when I go swimming, I don't feel pumped up to complete my usual number of laps. However, when I tell myself I'll hop into a jacuzzi for a few minutes after finishing my workout, it gets better as I know there's something nice waiting for me at the end of the session.

I don't need motivation at all to go climbing, but when I'm at the climbing gym, the vision of having a nice meal once I get back home – tired after a hard session – can give me additional energy to climb.

If there's a sauna at your gym, promise yourself a lazy session there once you finish your regular workout. If you're heading out for a run, tell yourself you can have a guilt-free binge session of watching your favorite TV series. If you're sore after your previous workout and don't feel like exercising again, tell yourself you'll get a massage – but only if you complete your workout for the day.

Ideally, come up with healthy rewards – or at least rewards that won't set you back. Going for an hourly run only to eat a huge piece of cake afterwards is not a good idea. Meeting with friends for some afternoon coffee after a 90-minute bike ride is better.

Listen to Music, Podcasts or Audiobooks

A 2012 study has shown that listening to music reduces the perception of effort while exercising with low to moderate intensity by ~10%[xxxix]. Additionally, listening to your favorite songs while exercising may reduce the resistance to engage in physical activity.

Podcasts or audiobooks can also be a good alternative to music if you enjoy listening to them. While they may not reduce the perception of effort, they'll make your workouts easier and possibly make you feel like the time flies by more quickly.

I usually dislike biking solo, but if I haven't been for a few days and can't find a partner, I download a few podcasts to my smartphone and listen to them while cycling. It makes the otherwise dull activity of biking alone more exciting.

Benefit from the Sunk Cost Fallacy

The sunk cost fallacy is the tendency to continue doing something once an investment in resources like money, effort, or time has been made – even when it's no longer rational to continue[xl]. In essence, it's throwing good money after bad.

For instance, people who have bought a non-refundable movie ticket will still go see the movie despite not really wanting to (because otherwise they would "waste" the money spent for the ticket).

While in most cases the sunk cost fallacy leads to irrational decisions and even more waste, you can use it to your benefit to stay motivated to exercise – just pay upfront for a 3-month, 6-month, or 12-month pass at the gym (or elsewhere) and let yourself fall victim to the fallacy so you'll have more motivation not to waste it.

I usually go swimming once a week. I don't find it as enjoyable as other activities (though I still like it), so a 3-month pass (despite being extremely cheap) gives me additional motivation to visit the pool at least once a week. I don't want to waste the money, even though skipping a few workouts would mean losing just a few bucks.

While this technique alone won't guarantee you'll stay motivated to exercise, it's just another tool that will help you stick to your resolutions, hopefully for long enough to develop a permanent habit.

HOW TO STAY MOTIVATED TO EXERCISE: QUICK RECAP

1. Setting goals – both performance-related goals as well as more general ones – will keep you motivated both in the beginning stages of learning a new sport as well as when practicing it for a few months or even a few years.

Make your goals Specific, Measurable, Achievable, Realistic, and Time-bound, but don't go crazy about it – if your primary reason for exercise is health and fitness, you don't have to track every single aspect of your performance. Set simple goals so you can track your progress and get motivated by it, not necessarily to become a world-class athlete.

2. In the case of being more experienced with a given sport, not only set new long-term goals, but also set goals that will lead to quick, visible improvements (usually related to things you don't practice often, but are a welcome change from the primary focus). These fun "side missions" will help you keep more enjoyment in your regular sessions.

3. Start a chain in your calendar and cross off days with a big red X each day you exercise. It sounds like a silly thing to do, but it can be enough to help you stay motivated until the habit of exercise becomes a permanent thing in your life.

4. Don't think in terms of "all or nothing" on your lazy days. If you can't make yourself go to the gym, put on your jogging shoes, or attend a yoga class, at least do an easy alternative – some bodyweight exercises at home, a brief walk, or a bout of dynamic stretching. It's better than nothing, and you'll reduce the risk of falling out of your habit completely.

5. Keep records of your workouts. Even noting it down on a piece of paper with a few words describing the session will be enough to keep track of your progress and increase your motivation to keep going as you see your progress.

6. Give yourself rewards for performing exercise – especially on the days you don't feel like doing it. Make sure that your rewards are beneficial to you, or

at least don't set you back fitness-wise. Think relaxation and enjoyment, not wild indulging.

7. Music can reduce the perception of effort while exercising. If you practice a certain type of activity by yourself, listening to music can be a good way to get yourself more excited about the workout and make it feel less strenuous. Alternatively, listen to podcasts or audiobooks.

8. The sunk cost fallacy (tendency to keep investing in things you've already invested in, even if it's no longer something you want to do) can help you stay motivated to exercise. Buy a long-term gym pass (or a pass for whichever place you visit to practice sports) and remind yourself of it next time you don't feel like working out. Your brain will irrationally trick you into thinking you're losing a lot by letting your pass go to waste. Consequently, you'll be more likely to use it.

Chapter 4: How to Enjoy Exercise

You'd like to start exercising, but you find it boring or you simply don't like it. But is it really always that dull? Do you always have to approach exercise as if it's unenjoyable – a chore to be done?

Not necessarily.

In this chapter we'll cover the most important tips how to start enjoying exercise so you no longer have to force yourself to do it, but can actually look forward to it. And it's simpler than you think. You just have to learn a few tricks to avoid the boring types of exercise and come up with physical activities that will get you addicted (in a good way).

Do This and Never Hate Exercising Again

"If your workout feels like work, it's not worth it," is a basic rule of thumb that will help you avoid the wrong kinds of exercise.

Granted, sometimes it takes more than one or two sessions to learn to enjoy a specific activity, but it's generally easy to say what feels like work and what feels like play. When in doubt, always choose play.

If you feel like the only reason you're doing a certain exercise is because it's good for you, it's actually bad for you. It can add a lot of stress in your life by introducing yet another obligation "for your own good." Exercise only ceases to be a burden and becomes an activity that improves the quality of your life if you like it and would do it willingly even if it didn't come with health benefits.

For this reason I stay away from all kinds of structured fitness classes where the focus is not on having fun and general sportsmanship, but on the general benefits of exercise.

A general rule is that if it doesn't have a simple name that most people immediately recognize and can picture what it's about, stay away from it – unless you genuinely find it fun.

"Fat burning exercises," "fitness classes for women 40+," "flat stomach fitness," or "shock fitness" are all examples of fitness classes that you'll probably find boring, or at least not particularly immersive. Yoga, tennis, basketball, or golf can all provide a never-ending source of inspiration and motivation to exercise because there's more to them than just burning your stomach fat.

If you enjoy structured fitness, that's great – keep doing it. If, however, you've always abhorred them, but felt it was your obligation to go to the local gym and take them because "hey, they're called 'flat stomach fitness' and that's what I want," give yourself a pass and stop.

No matter how long you keep taking these classes, they will never cease to be a challenge for your willpower and a reason to procrastinate. They can still provide results, but why make yourself suffer so much if you can opt for something more enjoyable instead?

Ask yourself what sounds or looks like fun – regardless of how silly or inappropriate for your age, gender, background, etc. – and do it.

Pole dancing fascinates you? Go and do it. Yes, even if you're a guy. You're not any less of a man because you choose it over pumping iron at the gym.

Krav maga sounds like something you'd do eagerly? You're no less of a woman if you choose to master this Israeli self-defense system instead of wearing a pink tank top and attending aerobic classes.

Throw away the stereotypes and go where the excitement is. Let others sweat their guts out doing exercises they hate while you move your body with a smile on your face.

I could list tons of ideas for sports here, but ultimately your final choice will depend on what's available in your area, how you can fit it in your schedule, whether it excites you, and whether you're physically capable of doing it.

9 Types of Non-Sport Physical Activity to Enjoy

Let's assume you can't find a sport you'd like to practice. Or you don't want to learn any sport specifically – all you want is to move your body in an enjoyable and healthy way. While I think that focusing on a specific sport is better because it gives you structure and an easy way to track your progress, that doesn't mean it's the only option.

Below are some physical activities that don't focus on a specific sport and are just some good ways to become physically active. Most of them require you to forget about being a big responsible adult and embrace a child-like spirit of play and exploration.

1. Go to a body of water

Go to the nearest body of water – a lake, ocean, sea, etc. – and spend an entire morning or afternoon there with a group of friends or family. Swim a little, wade, take a walk, or throw a Frisbee.

A few hours spent in such a way won't feel like exercise at all, while giving you plenty of opportunities to get your body moving.

2. Go hiking

If you're into beautiful scenery and exploring wilderness, few things are better than hiking. It allows you to benefit both from surrounding yourself with nature and from exercise.

Hikes that take a few hours provide well over the minimum amount of exercise you should get each week. Moreover, they exercise different parts of your muscles, especially when you're hiking in the mountains. Lastly, they don't feel like a boring set of exercises – and that's what we're after.

3. Keep up with a kid

If you've ever tried to keep up with a 5-year old kid, you know how much energy she has and how difficult it can be not to lose your breath when trying to participate in all of the games she invents.

Consequently, it's a perfect type of physical activity for every person who dislikes regular exercise. It doesn't feel like exercise – because it's not exercise, it's pure play. It also serves an important role of strengthening your bond with the kid, whether it's your niece, daughter, or your friend's child.

4. Play Twister

Please don't say it's reserved for kids. People of all ages can enjoy games of dexterity, and if you rarely engage in physical activity requiring balance and flexibility, Twister can be a great choice for you and your entire family or a group of friends.

5. Dance

Dancing is yet another way to engage in strenuous physical activity without it feeling like exercise. Try a traditional dance and not a dance fitness program like Zumba – that can feel more like boring fitness classes than dance and the art that's behind it.

It doesn't matter what type of a dance you practice as long as you enjoy it. A few hours of dancing a week – or a wild night out each week – will provide your body with enough exercise to feel like you've just finished a workout (while not feeling like exercise while doing it).

6. Get a dog

Dogs are perfect companions for long walks. A dog requires at least three to four walks a day, each at least 10-minute long, which in total translates to about twice the minimum amount of exercise you should get each week.

For even more activity, get a dog-friendly Frisbee to get a workout for your upper body, too. Don't feel silly chasing after the dog or playing with it.

7. Travel

Traveling can be a great way to get more exercise if you spend more time exploring the local attractions and not just exploring how comfortable the armchairs by the swimming pool are.

When in a different city or a foreign country, you'll probably tend to walk more and possibly engage in more sports and physical activity in general (for instance, hiking, or surfing lessons) just because enjoying the local places requires doing so (what's the attraction of riding a bus to Machu Picchu when compared with actually hiking the entire trail?).

8. Have sex

Please don't think about it in terms of exercise and calories burned while doing it. Sex is a natural, powerful way of bonding that can also provide some of the benefits of exercise.

A 2013 study on 21 couples compared the effects of moderate exercise on a treadmill and sex. The scientists found that sex is performed at a moderate intensity and "may potentially be considered, at times, as a significant exercise"[xli].

While sex isn't likely to become your primary way to exercise, next time you find yourself saying you don't have time for exercise, remind yourself that you can replace it with a different type of "workout" that will probably not be such a burden on your willpower.

9. Gardening and outdoor activities

Gardening, and especially doing things like yanking out weeds or raking by hand, is a calming, almost meditative-like activity that can not only help you reduce stress, but get you moving a little and get your muscles more active.

Other types of outdoor activities like splitting your own wood (instead of buying bundles of firewood) or fixing things around the house also count as low-intensity exercise.

Knife or hatchet throwing, skills that can be technically considered sports are also a good way to spend time outside in an active way and get a solid workout.

What If it's Not Fun?

Some types of exercise are necessary, or at least recommended to include in your workout schedule, yet not necessarily exciting. A good example in my case is static stretching that should be done after every single workout.

To make stretching more enjoyable, I try to find the little things I like about the activity – such as the feeling of my muscles stretching or an almost meditative experience of enduring the pain when it comes to more painful stretches.

If you struggle with exercises that you find necessary but not fun, try to discover all of the little ways you can make them more pleasant. Music can work here and so can doing a particular activity with a friend. When you combine all of these little things into one big thing, chances are you'll associate the otherwise unpleasant or boring activity with these small, enjoyable things.

While I don't find stretching fun and wouldn't do it if it wasn't necessary for injury prevention and overall flexibility, I do look forward to the calming experience of the post-workout stretching session (and especially the injury prevention benefits associated with it that allow me to enjoy my fun workouts more).

HOW TO ENJOY EXERCISE: QUICK RECAP

1. Structured fitness classes are a good way to learn how to dislike all types of physical activity and never look forward to them. As these types of activities usually focus on performing a specific exercise and engaging a specific set of muscles instead of fun and self-mastery, it's better to avoid them and pick something that has always appealed to you.

On the other hand, if you enjoy these classes, by all means continue them – the key is to find something you find fun, regardless what others think about it.

2. You don't have to practice a specific sport to engage in physical activity. There are at least nine ways to move your body while not performing a particular sport. These ideas include: going to a body of water, hiking, keeping up with a kid, playing dexterity games like Twister, dancing, playing with or walking a dog, traveling, having sex, and gardening or other types of outdoor activities.

3. If you need to perform a specific type of activity but don't look forward to it, make it more enjoyable by either discovering the little pleasant things about it (for instance, the calming feeling of stretching your muscles) or making the experience more bearable by listening to your favorite music or doing it with a friend.

Chapter 5: How to Improve Recovery, Prevent Injuries, and Handle Muscle Soreness

Perhaps you've been exercising for a year or two and you're struggling due to low energy, soreness, or burnout. Or each time you start a new workout routine your body gets so sore you don't want to exercise again, and then you go back to your old ways.

A common reason why people stop exercising is soreness, injuries, or pain associated with physical activity. In fact, the physical discomfort is probably the most challenging part of introducing an exercise habit for people used to a sedentary lifestyle.

After all, it's relatively easy to get off your couch and have your first session of exercise, but it gets much more difficult once you wake up the next day and every single muscle in your body feels like it's fried.

If you're starting out, muscle soreness is a guarantee. An injury – even a little one that heals in a few days – is also a possibility for an untrained body. It can deter you from your next session of exercise, thus breaking your chain. Unfortunately, the more time you take off, the more likely it will be you'll get sore yet again after your next workout.

DOMS (delayed onset muscle soreness) can't be avoided if you haven't been exercising for a long time. However, according to Brad Schoenfeld and Bret Contreras and contrary to what some people think, experiencing muscle soreness after a training session isn't a good indicator of whether your exercise was effective or not[xlii].

In other words, don't fall into the trap of thinking that if you feel sore, you've had a good workout – it's a twisted way of thinking that can make you associate fitness with pain, which will lead to problems with willpower. Additionally, it can lead to an injury – and that will make sticking to your new habit impractical or even impossible.

While DOMS can't be avoided entirely, you can reduce its severity. As for the injuries, most risks can be eliminated by following some simple tips. Consequently, you'll reduce the risk of creating additional barriers to your habit of exercise.

Since it's hard to study DOMS or recovery and provide conclusive evidence about possible therapies, the eight ideas below are only suggestions to try and not sure-fire ways that work for everyone. Still, try them next time you feel sore and you'll possibly reduce your resistance to the next workout.

1. Foam rolling

Since self-myofascial release (targeted muscle tension release) is an emerging form of therapy, there's still not enough conclusive scientific evidence regarding it (for instance, available studies were done on just a few participants).

However, a 2015 systematic review suggests that foam rolling may be effective as both a pre- and post-workout way to reduce muscle soreness[xliii]. Another

2015 systematic review also suggests that foam rolling can enhance recovery[xliv] and make it easier on your willpower to keep exercising.

A 2015 Canadian study on foam rolling and DOMS has shown that 20 minutes of foam rolling after exercise (immediately after, 24 hours after, and 48 hours after) reduced DOMS in 8 participants when measured by sprint time, power, and dynamic strength-endurance[xlv]. It's by no means ultimate proof that it will work for you, but it's a good idea to test it as you can only gain from it.

If you'd like to test how foam rolling works on your body, invest in a foam roller and watch a few instructional videos on YouTube on how to use it. Then foam roll after each workout session and ideally, the following two days, too (that's when your muscles will be the most sore).

Please keep in mind that foam rolling will be painful, especially during the first few weeks when you'll have to deal with all of the accumulated tensions in your entire body. However, releasing tension and relaxing your muscles will help you feel better in general, thus making it easier to exercise.

At the time of writing this book, I've been using my foam roller religiously three times a week for about two years. I find it an extremely helpful tool for reducing tension in my back and calves, which helps me perform better during my workouts as well as reduce the risk of injuries.

2. Get a massage

Massage has been found effective at alleviating DOMS, but not at improving muscle function. In other words, it's useful for the psychological benefits of reduced soreness, but won't improve your body's physical recovery.

A 2003 study showed that massage performed two hours after exercise didn't improve hamstring function but reduced the intensity of soreness 48 hours post-exercise[xlvi].

Another study in 2005 determined that a 10-minute sports massage 3 hours after exercise was effective in alleviating DOMS by approximately 30%. It was also helpful in reducing swelling[xlvii].

Yet another 2005 paper concluded that "Post-exercise massage has been shown to reduce the severity of muscle soreness but massage has no effects on muscle functional loss"[xlviii].

Finally, a 2013 review on the effects of massage therapy on DOMS has shown inconclusive evidence in the same vein – massage can help with soreness, but not performance enhancement[xlix].

If you're just starting out with your exercise habit, it's possible that soreness will pose a barrier for you to exercise again in two or three days. If you feel like experimenting, have a massage (deep sports massage, not the regular relaxing light massage) on the muscles that were the most active during your bout of exercise. Even if it doesn't help with physical recovery, it should help reduce soreness – and that, in turn, will make it a bit easier to exercise again.

3. Drink coffee or tea

Surprisingly, caffeine is good not only for turning zombies into people in the morning, but also for reducing muscle soreness.

A 2013 study has shown that ingesting caffeine immediately before upper-body resistance training enhances performance. Moreover, sustained caffeine ingestion in the days after the exercise decreased the perception of soreness[l].

Turns out you have yet another good reason to keep drinking coffee or tea. Granted, caffeine pills will most likely work better than drinking tea or coffee, but a much more pleasant drink should still help by not only giving you more energy for the workout, but also reducing the pain after it.

4. Get proper nutrients

Studies on small sample sizes suggest that proper nutrition can help with recovery as well as muscle soreness.

For instance, a 2006 study on 17 men showed that amino acid supplementation reduces exercise-associated muscle strength loss[li].

A 2010 study on 12 women has confirmed the same findings that muscle damage may be suppressed by BCAA supplementation prior to exercise[lii].

The simplest way to get amino acids shortly before exercise is to consume BCAA's (branched chain amino acids). They can be bought in capsule or powder form in every store with supplements (and most likely in your gym, too).

Antioxidants are another part of the puzzle. They reduce excessive inflammation, thus promoting recovery and reducing pain.

A 1996 paper on the role of antioxidant vitamins and enzymes in the prevention of exercise-induced muscle damage states outright that "the question whether antioxidant vitamins and antioxidant enzymes play a protective role in exercise-induced muscle damage can be answered affirmatively. The human studies reviewed indicate that antioxidant vitamin supplementation can be recommended to individuals performing regular heavy exercise"[liii].

A 2012 study on blueberries and exercise-induced muscle damage has shown that a blueberry smoothie prior to and after exercise accelerates recovery of muscle peak isometric strength.

There are also studies covering the beneficial recovery-boosting effects of cherry juice.

In one British study, drinking 12 fl oz (0.35 l) of cherry juice twice a day for eight days has been found to decrease some of the symptoms of exercise induced muscle damage[liv].

Another study in 2011 agrees, showing that Montmorency cherry juice reduces muscle damage caused by intensive strength exercise[lv].

Yet another study in 2010 on tart cherry juice following marathon running has also confirmed the same findings. As the scientists noted: "The cherry juice appears to provide a viable means to aid recovery following strenuous exercise by increasing total anti-oxidative capacity, reducing inflammation, lipid peroxidation and so aiding in the recovery of muscle function"[lvi].

Last but not least, a 2010 American study has shown that ingesting tart cherry juice for 7 days prior to and during a strenuous running event can minimize post-run muscle pain[lvii].

All of these studies suggest that foods rich in antioxidant and anti-inflammatory properties may help reduce muscle damage and pain during strenuous exercise. Stock up on berries and tart cherry juice, consume them prior to and after exercising, and you'll suffer less after your first workouts and have more willpower to continue.

5. Warm-up, stretch, cool down

It's important to precede each exercise session with a proper warm-up (pre-workout) and follow it with a cool-down routine of exercises like jumping jacks, stationary bike, jogging, etc. The goal of a warm-up is to get your body ready for the exercise and reduce the risk of injuries. The objective of a cool-down is to help your body transition from exercise to rest.

A 2007 paper has shown that you should perform a warm-up and a stretching protocol within the 15 minutes prior to physical activity to receive the most benefit and deter injuries[lviii].

A 2010 meta-analysis on 32 studies determined that a warm-up improves performance in 79% of the criterions examined and that "there is little evidence to suggest that warming-up is detrimental to sports participants.[lix]" While more well-conducted studies are needed to prove the beneficial role of a warm-up, it's safe to say a warm-up is as necessary as every sports coach will tell you.

There are two types of stretching, both of which are necessary for injury prevention as well as improving recovery and minimizing muscle pain.

The first type is static stretching, the one you're probably more familiar with – holding a stretch for 30 to 90 seconds, usually with a burning feeling in the muscles being stretched.

This type of stretching should only be done after your workouts, and never before them because it can impair strength by causing joint instability[lx]. A 2013 meta-analysis has concluded that the usage of static stretching as the sole activity during warm-up routine should generally be avoided due to reduced strength, power, and explosive performance[lxi].

Static stretching – when done after a workout – is beneficial for recovery and strength increases, but not necessarily for DOMS (a 2011 meta-analysis suggests it doesn't reduce DOMS at all[lxii]).

As former Soviet Special Forces physical training instructor Pavel Tsatsouline writes in his article, "The benefits of stretching are enormous. Stretching can increase your strength by 10%. It is a lot. The man [Russian Master of Sports Alexander Faleev] explains that 'when you lift a weight your muscles contract. And after the workout the muscles remain contracted for some time. The following restoration of the muscles' length is what recovery is. Until the muscle has restored its length, it has not recovered. Hence he who does not stretch his muscles slows down the recuperation process and retards his gains.' Besides, tension and relaxation are two sides of the same coin, 'if the muscle forgets how to lengthen, it will contract more poorly. And that is stagnation of strength'"[lxiii].

I learned my lesson about the power of static stretching when my manual therapist recommended I start doing it after each climbing session for the pain in my finger joints and feet (both common among beginning climbers) and for general injury prevention for the entire body. After just a week, I noticed a considerable decrease in pain and greatly improved overall flexibility when climbing. Three weeks later, the pain was almost non-existent. I've been a believer ever since.

The second type of stretching is dynamic stretching, also called ballistic stretching. You should do this type before exercise along with a warm-up. Unlike static stretching, a 2008 study found dynamic stretching improves power, strength, muscular endurance, anaerobic capacity, and agility performance[lxiv].

Once I started putting more focus on dynamic stretching and warm-ups before my climbing sessions, I reduced the occurrence of little pains when climbing and enjoyed greater flexibility, too.

Explaining how to perform static or dynamic stretches goes beyond the scope of this book. A quick YouTube search will provide you with all the routines you need for proper pre- and post-workout stretching.

6. Go to a sauna

A 2015 Thai and Malaysian study has shown that visiting a sauna before exercise can help reduce delayed onset muscle soreness of the wrist extensors[lxv]. These findings are consistent with general advice that if you want to treat muscle soreness, increasing blood flow to the muscles and subsequent increased oxygen delivery may help you feel better.

Sports medicine specialist David Geier says in an article on saunas and recovery that a sauna "causes you to sweat and can help release endorphins. And the heat also increases blood flow to the muscle and the periphery of the body, which probably does help sore muscles feel better temporarily."

He also points out that while sitting in a sauna is not a good idea after a workout – sitting in a sauna for more than five minutes is a form of passive exercise that will delay the recovery process – spending a few minutes in a sauna before your workout is a better idea because it "may indeed help you feel warmed up and relieve some immediate muscle pain"[lxvi].

To sum up, while a post-workout sauna probably won't help much long-term, it will make you feel better temporarily and can prepare you psychologically for the next workout. For the most benefit, consider a few minutes in a sauna before exercising.

7. Sleep

Proper recovery can't happen without high-quality sleep. Numerous studies have shown that sleep loss – and especially chronic sleep loss[lxvii] – negatively affects human performance to a great extent[lxviii, lxix].

A 2014 review has shown that sleep deprivation can have "significant effects on athletic performance, especially submaximal, prolonged exercise. Compromised sleep may also influence learning, memory, cognition, pain perception, immunity and inflammation"[lxx].

There's no question that sleep is a mandatory part of a proper recovery regimen. Ideally, you should sleep enough hours every single day, and not try to catch up on sleep on the weekends. Recovery sleep during the weekend won't magically eliminate all of the symptoms of lack of sleep[lxxi] as more time is needed to fix long-term sleep deprivation.

What's interesting, lack of sleep may increase pain sensitivity for both acute pain (lasting less than 3 to 6 months) and chronic pain[lxxii]. If you suffer from an injury or have any chronic pain, you should pay even more attention to getting enough sleep.

As for the amount of sleep you should get, it all depends on how you feel. After particularly exhausting days (swimming, tennis, and climbing all during the same day) I sleep for up to 10 hours or more if I feel I need it. I don't berate myself in the morning for not waking up early enough. The two additional hours I could "gain" if I woke up earlier would extend my recovery time while also reducing my general sense of well-being and performance.

8. Exercise again

Last but not least, the news you probably don't want to hear: one of the best ways to reduce DOMS is to exercise again.

Exercise-induced hypoalgesia (increased pain thresholds and pain tolerance thanks to exercise) has been proven to occur in endurance training in sports like running, cycling, and swimming[lxxiii]. If you suffer from muscle soreness, going on a bike ride, jogging, or having a swim can temporarily help soothe the pain.

Whenever I suffer from DOMS, I usually exercise more despite the pain. You won't feel the pain while exercising nearly as much as you expect, and the soreness will be greatly reduced after the workout.

Please keep in mind you don't have to engage your muscles with the same intensity as the day before. Light exercise – even if it's just a simple walk for leg soreness – will help.

When Common Knowledge Can Actually Reduce Your Willpower

Many athletes take cold showers, use contrast therapy (by alternating between hot and cold showers) or immerse themselves in cold water to improve recovery or reduce DOMS. It's possible you follow this advice, too, and unknowingly reduce your willpower by using this therapy for the wrong application.

Science hasn't found solid evidence that either of these methods alone is enough to reduce DOMS to a noticeable effect. In fact, more and more studies emerge stating that cold therapy only provides a placebo effect while negatively affecting performance.

A 2015 Japanese study uncovered that the group of participants that used cooling after exercise experienced significantly lower increases or no increases in strength, muscle diameter, and endurance when compared to the non-cooled group[lxxiv].

In other words, listening to common advice can actually make you weaker next time you exercise and then discourage you from working out.

Some studies suggest that there's a possibility that such therapies can – to a very small, statistically insignificant extent – help with self-reported recovery (and not objective measures like increased strength)[lxxv].

A 2010 French study shows that whole-body cryotherapy after severe exercise can help[lxxvi], though I can't see most people looking for a nearby cryotherapy chamber immediately after a workout to stand for three minutes in -166°F (-110°C) just to improve your recovery a bit.

As sports medicine doctor Gabe Mirkin says, "About all icing is good for is a placebo effect"[lxxvii]. If anecdotal evidence convinces you, a simple therapy with cold showers or ice packs may be worth trying, if only for improved perception of your own wellbeing or a placebo effect (hey, it still helps, right?).

A 2010 Singaporean research paper says, "a holistic approach to recovery will give a better response rather than an isolated recovery technique"[lxxviii]. If cold therapy makes you feel good and helps you keep motivation to exercise despite soreness, by all means continue it.

However, according to professor of exercise science David Pascoe at Auburn University, if you're after maximum strength, it's better to skip it[lxxix]. As he says, "If athletes feel pretty sore, then get into a tub, and come out feeling great, they're going to have a better workout. That might be enough to consider icing if you aren't worried about muscle and strength gains."

If, however, you know that reduced gains will decrease your motivation, focus on a more holistic approach of doing proper warm-ups, stretching, following other suggested pre-workout ways to reduce DOMS, and simply exercising despite soreness.

Please note, though, that what we've covered applies only to the effects of cold therapy on recovery and DOMS, not the other health benefits they can provide (like pain relief in case of injuries).

How to Take a Break without Destroying Your Habit

Common sense would make you think that when you'd compare a person training 52 weeks a year with a person training 16–24 weeks a year, the former would be much stronger than the latter. Yet, as fitness coach Jason Feruggia and any strength coach would tell you, the strength gains aren't that much different in either of these cases, and the athletes resting for longer can actually experience greater gains[lxxx].

Consequently, breaks are good for you and can help you achieve the same or better results with less effort – given that you're able to get back into your routine after taking a break. And herein lies the biggest problem – how do you resume a habit of exercise if you've been taking it easy for a week or two, or even an entire month in the case of a forced break due to an illness or an injury?

The most important thing you should remember is to never truly stop exercising at all. Complete physical inactivity has a way of promoting laziness that's hard to escape once the break is over.

If you're forced to take a break and have to give up all kinds of exercise due to an illness or an injury, at least try to move a little – as much as your doctor allows you to. If you're taking a break to recover, stop for a week or two with your regular, most strenuous exercises, but keep doing other, low-intensity exercises like taking walks, cycling, etc.

Every twelve weeks, I take a week or two off and don't lift weights. These breaks greatly reduce the amount of exercise I get, but they only serve as a recovery tool for me – they don't cause any problems once I restart my routine. Taking a break from the gym doesn't mean I stop exercising at all. I only pause my weightlifting sessions to let my body recover while I still practice other sports, albeit usually with lower intensity.

In addition, these breaks serve another important purpose – they help me stay motivated to lift weights by preventing general psychological and physical burnout and/or injuries that have a higher chance of happening if you're over-trained.

If you still maintain some kind of a fitness routine during a break – even if it's just a few walks a week – it's still enough to help you resume your previous routine once you're ready.

What if going back to your old routine means experiencing the old problems you're not looking forward to, like sore muscles and general reluctance to exercise even if you know you'll enjoy it once you get back into it?

In such a case, start slow and gradually increase intensity until you feel you're back to your previous shape and mindset. When I return to the gym after my week-long break, I don't start with the weights I lifted the last time I was at the gym. I reduce the intensity by 10%, which still makes training feel like a solid workout, but not so challenging that I'm unable to move my body the next day.

The same advice applies to other types of sports. If you go on 2-hour long bike rides four times a week and take a 14-day break from cycling, don't start with four 2-hour long sessions a week when you go back. Take it easier by starting with two or three 90-minute sessions the first week. It will make it easier for your body to re-accustom to your previous routine, thus reducing the soreness and general reluctance to exercise.

It's a good idea to develop your own recovery system and stick to it religiously. For instance, I always take a week-long break from the gym every three months. In addition to that, I make sure to increase the number of days recovering from other sports (like climbing) whenever I feel I have low energy. Just one additional day of rest can have huge effects on your overall motivation, thus helping you stick with your fitness routine permanently.

However, don't fall into the trap of taking breaks on a whim. Plan them in advance so you avoid taking emotionally-dictated breaks just because you don't feel like exercising on a given day. Such a behavior can lead to destroying your habit and reducing motivation.

Last but not least, don't feel guilty about taking a break. As long as you take it weeks or months after you develop a permanent habit of exercise (and not the first time you face obstacles), they won't hurt and can only help.

HOW TO IMPROVE RECOVERY, PREVENT INJURIES, AND HANDLE MUSCLE SORENESS: QUICK RECAP

1. If you start exercising, muscle soreness is a guarantee. There's also a higher risk of an injury, especially if your body is not used to exercise at all. Consequently, it pays to learn and use different ways to manage DOMS, improve recovery, and prevent injuries.

Post-workout foam rolling is an effective way to reduce delayed onset muscle soreness as well as prevent injuries. Sports massage is also helpful, but only serves psychological soreness-reducing benefits. Drinking caffeine has been proven to decrease the perception of soreness, too.

Proper nutrition can also promote recovery as well as reduce pain after the exercise. Getting essential amino acids in the form of BCAA's can help, and so can anti-oxidant rich inflammation-reducing foods like blueberries or tart cherry juice.

Dynamic stretching before workouts help with performance and reduces the risk of injuries, while static stretching after workouts help optimize recovery. Don't forget about the proper warm-up and cool down routines as they help your body get ready for exercise (or help it transition from exercise to rest) and prevent injuries.

Going to a sauna after a workout is another strategy that can help you reduce soreness and feel better, though it mostly provides temporary psychological effects. For an additional pain-reducing and warming-up dose, consider a short 5-minute session in a sauna prior to exercise.

Don't forget that recovery – both physical and psychological – can't happen without high-quality sleep.

Lastly, one of the most effective ways to deal with soreness and help your body recover more quickly is to exercise again. Even a low-intensity walk can help reduce soreness.

2. A popular cold therapy for improving recovery and reducing DOMS can actually be detrimental to your performance during the next workout, thus making it more probable you'll give up exercising.

Studies are inconclusive, but they suggest that ice for DOMS only provides a placebo effect and makes sense only for psychological benefits and not for maximum strength and endurance.

3. When taking a break from exercise, don't stop exercising altogether. Try to have some physical activity so that when you resume your routine, you won't dramatically increase the amount of exercise you get immediately.

Regular breaks – when not taken on a whim and planned in advance before developing injuries or burnout – can help you stay motivated to exercise for years to come. Don't feel guilty about taking them. When done properly, they'll only help you progress.

Chapter 6: On Other Exercise-Related Issues

There are many issues related with exercise that I've only covered partly in the previous chapters or that I haven't covered at all before, but are important parts of the equation for creating a lifelong habit of exercise.

In this chapter, we'll talk about how to deal with other people and their approach to exercise or their approach to you exercising. Support (or its lack thereof) can make or break your fitness plans, and it's important to know how to deal with this problem.

Secondly, we'll talk about managing your expectations (setting the wrong ones will discourage you from exercise), and handle the problem of self-criticism, discomfort and low self-esteem when exercising.

Lastly, we'll cover the seasons and how they affect exercise habits (and what to do to stick to your habit despite harsh winters).

How to Deal with Other People

As mentioned briefly in the prologue, a study in 2009 found lack of support is the number one barrier to exercise, beating out lack of willpower. This means that other people can make or break your resolutions, and their influence has a lot to do with how you look and feel.

In the most common scenario, when you start exercising, one or more of your unhelpful, physically inactive friends (or family members) starts poking fun at you or displaying her resistance to your change in a variety of other ways. This essentially communicates "don't you dare change your life for the better." If you do, it will be obvious she's unable (or unwilling) to make such changes herself.

While there are dozens of different ways to deal with this problem, the one piece of advice I've found the most useful is to focus on yourself and ignore what others are saying.

It all comes down to trusting yourself and your decisions. If you know that exercise will change your life for the better, why on earth would you let others influence you to stop improving? Because of fear of being judged by them?

Now, I don't believe that you should be a lone wolf trying to change your life without any support whatsoever. Ignoring others and trusting yourself is the first step. The second step is surrounding yourself with people who share your attitude.

Fortunately, when you start exercising, it will be extremely easy to make friends with other people who either want to change their lives or have already changed them.

In the climbing gym I attend, you can meet a wide variety of people. A vast majority of them share one thing – they love climbing and support others who share their passion.

Whether you're a 40-year old single mom, a 25-year old overweight student, or a 55-year old man with a belly, most will be happy to give you advice, guidance, and support so you can learn the sport. Friendships happen naturally when you're both trying to do the same bouldering problem or try to scale the same climbing route.

Things aren't different in other venues populated by sports enthusiasts. If you go to a fitness gym, both the staff and fellow gym goers will help you. If you want to learn how to dance, other passionate dancers will be there to support you.

If a lack of support bothers you a lot, choosing a sport that can be practiced with others will make it easier to befriend people who will support you (and help you ignore the people who aren't helpful).

Whenever possible, finding an ally in a friend or a family member is better, but if it's not possible, look around and make new friends. There's no rule prohibiting you from making new supportive friends when learning a new sport.

Alternatively, consider joining a forum dedicated to fitness or the sport you want to learn. You could also find a fitness social network (or utilize the ones you already use for following and interacting with fitness-oriented people).

A lot of knowledge and inspiration for the sports I've practiced so far came from online interactions – both in the passive form by reading the posts and articles of other people as well as in a more direct way of personal messages and seeking personal advice.

Please keep in mind that many people online try to provide well-intentioned advice but don't have a lot of experience themselves. On forums, high post counts and reputation can help identify whose advice is valuable and whose is not. On social networks it can be more difficult to verify, though usually you can trust the most active users who provide thorough advice.

No matter the experience, all people – both beginners and experts – in such places can give you support to continue working out. Many forums offer the ability to create a progress thread that works in the same way as a public journal of your efforts. If you don't mind divulging a bit of information about yourself online, consider setting up your own progress thread so you can get personal advice from other people and become an inspiration for others.

How to Manage Your Expectations

When you start exercising, it's possible you'll set unrealistic expectations for yourself or compare yourself with others, thus losing motivation to work out. To avoid these problems from influencing your habit, take two steps.

The first step is to learn about the realistic goals specific to what you're doing. Set your goals according to this information and avoid assuming that you'll beat the odds. If you do better, great. If not, you didn't expect to anyway, so it won't ruin your resolve.

For instance, a beginner to weightlifting may assume he'll be able to bench press 200 pounds (91 kg) within six months. However, a quick look at realistic fitness goals shows that the average male needs up to two years of training to be able to bench press 1.2x his body weight[lxxxi].

When the unrealistic beginner realizes he's still far away from reaching his goal, he may be tempted to give up. After all, in his mind, he has failed and wasted six months of his life – notwithstanding he had made great progress in line with what he could have realistically accomplished during this time.

Whenever starting to learn a new sport, seek out what goals you can set for yourself and educate yourself about the realities of it.

Most sports look much easier while you're watching them than when you try them. This is because people with a lot of experience tend to make things look easy, but that's only because they've been repeating the same moves over and over again for years on end. It's precisely their experience that makes it look easy, and not the sport itself.

Unfortunately, this makes it easy to overestimate how long it's going to take to master them. Remember this and find goals suitable for beginners so you don't get frustrated.

The second step – the step to avoid comparing yourself with others – is related to those experienced people. Become more aware of your abilities and your limits, and then judge your performance only in relation to them, not other people. In other words, if you feel you've pushed yourself to the limits, blaming yourself for not being as good as others makes no sense. As long as you're venturing outside of your comfort zone to grow and make progress, it's all that matters.

In climbing, routes can be done in a wide variety of ways. A 6' 1" tall (186 cm) man can easily reach a handhold a 5' 6" tall (167 cm) female wouldn't be able to reach without having to find another foothold before reaching the same handhold.

Why would she berate herself for not being able to finish the route if she has an entirely different set of advantages and drawbacks when climbing? As long as she's doing all she can to climb the route, losing motivation because a much taller man did it without any problems is ridiculous.

Focus on yourself, your abilities, and your limits, and let the others do their thing.

Put an End to Self-Criticism

Doubts and self-criticism can discourage you from ever trying to make changes in your life for the fear you'll fail or make a fool out of yourself. Fortunately, you can fix these problems as neither self-doubt nor self-criticism are lifelong sentences that will forever deter you from bettering yourself through exercise.

The three most common reasons for self-criticism when thinking about exercise are:

1. Pessimism

Long-term physical inactivity can lead to thoughts like "Who am I fooling? I'll never be able to exercise." It's nothing but pessimism reinforced by years of unsuccessful tries or intentions you never acted upon.

As much as I would love to give you a foolproof way to solve this problem, pessimism never disappears overnight and takes consistent practice, self-awareness, and willingness to make changes to develop a more positive outlook.

There are a few things that can help, though:

a. Support

If people around you are pessimistic, they won't help you fix your negative attitude. If, on the other hand, you can find support in people close to you and be open to their positive influence, they'll help you escape the trap of pessimism.

b. Gratitude

Expressing grateful thoughts on a daily basis, especially when related to your health and fitness, will help you break through the layer of pessimism.

When you start exercising, you can experience gratitude that you were able to have a 30-minute walk without struggling to catch your breath or do five laps in a swimming pool without a break. These positive thoughts – instead of berating yourself for how weak you are – will help you associate exercise with feeling good instead of feeling guilty for letting yourself go the past few years.

c. Positive surroundings and habits

In addition to surrounding yourself with positive people, make sure to eliminate all kinds of negative stimuli from your environment. For example, I don't read news nor visit any sites whose only objective is to make you feel negative. I also stay away from negative behaviors and habits like complaining, worrying, making yourself feel like a victim, etc.

You're most likely well aware of what websites, places, habits, and other stimuli make you feel negative. It can be a news site, a fitness magazine that tells you that you're never thin enough, your habit of worrying or complaining, or a local fitness gym where newcomers are met with skepticism. If it's something with a positive alternative, find it.

Make sure that what surrounds you is what builds you up instead of dragging you down. All these little changes, when combined, will support you to give up negativity and focus on the bright side of life, thus helping you introduce a habit of exercise in your life (that will further develop your optimism).

2. Low self-efficacy

Self-efficacy refers to the belief in your abilities to succeed in a specific situation[lxxxii]. You can have high self-efficacy for, say, knitting, and low self-efficacy for exercise. As long as your belief in your ability to exercise is low, it will be difficult to persist when faced with obstacles. It will be tricky to maintain your routine and will put limits on what you can accomplish.

In my book, *Confidence: How to Overcome Your Limiting Beliefs and Achieve Your Goals*, I talk about the Galatea effect[lxxxiii], a type of self-fulfilling prophecy that makes your self-expectations largely determine your performance.

If you have high self-expectations, you'll enjoy high performance. If you don't expect much from yourself, your performance will suffer, most likely leading to a drop in motivation and failure.

I go deep into the science and practical advice for developing self-efficacy in the aforementioned book. For the purposes of this book, the most crucial piece of advice to build self-efficacy is to ensure small wins.

The strategy of setting tiny goals and achieving them while constantly pushing the boundaries further and further will help you develop more belief in yourself, which will lead to better performance and less feelings of self-criticism and discouragement.

The smaller and easier the initial goals, the more likely it is you'll continue with your routine until it's a well-oiled machine.

For instance, if you want to start swimming but you're afraid you'll start drowning and embarrass yourself, start treading water in a shallow pool first. Remind yourself how it feels to swim (if you know how to swim, but haven't tried it for a long time), and each subsequent workout try to introduce a more challenging thing to try.

During the first few weeks, don't try anything that has a high chance of a failure as it can decrease your self-efficacy. After a streak of small wins you'll be less susceptible to discouragement because of one failure.

If you don't know how to swim at all, find an instructor or attend swimming classes aimed at complete beginners. The right teacher is aware that water can make people feel insecure and overly nervous and will lead you by the hand to build your self-efficacy tiny step by step.

If you don't feel you're ready for classes, get used to the swimming pool by simply treading water. Use a kickboard and other floatation aids to reduce your fear and gradually get used to what it's like to be in the water. If you continue with such a routine for a few weeks, your fear will eventually diminish, allowing you to consider swimming classes.

3. Low self-esteem

Low self-esteem is different than self-efficacy because while self-efficacy refers to specific beliefs about your abilities, self-esteem relates to your general evaluation of yourself. A more telling synonym of the word "self-esteem" is "self-respect" because that's what it comes down to in the end – low self-esteem means you have little respect for yourself.

How are you supposed to take care of your body if you care so little for your entire being? Some common tendencies of people with low self-esteem include:

- criticizing themselves for everything. Self-criticism makes it challenging to introduce any new habit because you'll constantly get angry at yourself for being so [fill in the blank].

- hypersensitivity to criticism and excessive will to please others. If you have friends who aren't physically active, they'll try to make you give up your goal to become fitter and probably succeed if you can't bear people criticizing you.

- chronic indecision, fear of failure and/or mistakes, and perfectionism. All of them will paralyze you when trying to introduce a habit of exercise.

Do you want to turn into a person with high self-esteem? Become aware of your current thought patterns, behaviors, and habits, and remodel them one by one to resemble the person you want to become.

In the past, I too suffered from low self-esteem. For me, it was a long process of self-discovery and changing my entire identity one block at a time.

First attempts at exercise (while I still thought I was a fitness failure because I was always one of the worst students during my physical exercise classes), first attempts to think in a more positive way (while I was still used to complaining every single hour of the day and having suicidal thoughts), and first attempts to exhibit a more confident behavior (while I was still paralyzed with fear among strangers, particularly women) were all the stepping stones on which I built the entire new foundation.

I can't sum up my story in a few paragraphs, and it would be a disservice to you to simplify it to such an extent.

Out of all the people with low self-esteem I've known, each had to take his or her own journey of self-discovery. These journeys usually took years before becoming firmly established in the mind. What each person had in common, though, is that he or she started – despite fear, self-criticism, perfectionism, indecision, and resentment.

NLP (an approach to communication and personal development) – particularly Tony Robbins' books, *Unlimited Power* and *Awaken the Giant Within* – contains countless powerful techniques for self-change that go far beyond the scope of this book and will help you on your journey toward high self-esteem.

Dealing with Seasons

If you live in a place with distinct seasons, harsh winter conditions can discourage you from exercising.

I stop biking altogether in the fall and winter because I dislike doing it when I feel cold. In-season, I go on bike rides at least 2-3 times a week. Consequently, off-season means a lot of lost exercise time due to the weather.

Consequently, I then shift to indoor physical activities. I can spend more time at the climbing gym, swim more, and play more tennis indoors. If the weather is good, I still like to get some exercise outside (long walks can still be enjoyable even if it's cold), but it's no longer the primary source of physical activity for me.

If you started exercising in, say, June, and by October you would stop biking because of the weather, there would be a high chance you would lose your new habit. Three to six months of reduced physical activity is a lot, even for a person who has a strong habit of exercise.

When considering which sports to practice, don't forget to have at least one sport that can be done indoors (and no, chess doesn't count). It doesn't mean you have to do it indoors during the summer, though – playing tennis outside on a warm, sunny day is always better than doing it inside. The benefits of physical exercise are not only about the exercise itself, but also about getting plenty of sunshine and enjoying the nice weather outside whenever possible.

ON OTHER EXERCISE-RELATED ISSUES: QUICK RECAP

1. Other people can make or break your resolutions, but only if you let them. If you have a friend or a family member who's unsupportive and criticizes you or pokes fun at you for trying to change your habits, counteract his or her negative influence with positive and supportive friends.

If you don't have any friends who can support you, pick a sport that's usually practiced with other people. This is an easy way to get to know other individuals who will support you.

Alternatively, seek support online. Frequenting forums or social networks populated with other fitness-oriented people will provide you with numerous opportunities to get advice, inspiration, and possibly develop new friendships.

2. Setting unrealistic expectations will make it difficult to stick to your new resolutions. Whenever starting a new sport, learn about the realistic goals you can achieve and avoid falling into the trap of thinking you're special and will beat the average. If

you do, that's great. But if not, it shouldn't deter you from exercising just because you couldn't achieve something very few people are able to do.

To avoid comparing yourself with others, focus on your abilities and your limits. As long as you make an effort to step outside your own comfort zone and do all you can to improve, you're on the right track.

Don't forget that comparing yourself with other people who have different bodies, skills, past experience with sports, etc. makes little sense because there are too many variables influencing the performance.

3. Pessimism, low self-efficacy, and low self-esteem can all make you prone to self-criticism.

If you want to deal with pessimism, consider paying more attention to the people, habits, behaviors, and places you surround yourself with as well as expressing more gratitude in your life.

To develop more self-efficacy for exercise, focus on achieving small wins that will slowly but surely build up your beliefs and help you lower resistance to take up bigger challenges.

Dealing with low self-esteem usually takes a few long years. However, the first step is always the same – it all starts with doing what a person with high self-esteem would do despite feeling apprehensive about it. Remodeling your default responses, habits, thought patterns, and behaviors will all help if you develop more awareness of the self-esteem-reducing tendencies you cultivate in your life so you can eliminate them.

4. If you live in a place with cold winters that make it hard or impossible to exercise outside, don't forget to have at least one option for exercising indoors. Don't make the mistake of exercising in the spring, summer, and fall and then taking it easy for the winter because it's almost guaranteed you won't be able to go back to your old habit when the next season comes.

Epilogue

Most people will need a few tries to establish a permanent habit of exercise. You'll have to try a few different sports, get discouraged more than a couple of times, and keep figuring things out until you come up with a routine that works for you. Perhaps you'll also have to re-wire some of your thoughts or behaviors and act despite indecision or perfectionism.

However, it will all be more than worth it. A strong habit of exercise will not only provide you with a myriad of health benefits, but also increase the quality of your life in general. You'll feel happier, more productive, and less prone to negative emotions.

Without doubt, exercise can change your life – as it has changed mine. Rest assured that few, if any, changes in your life will reward you with bigger benefits than consistently working out and using your body in as many (fun) ways as possible.

As a final reminder – a take-home message if you will – here are the five most important guidelines to introduce more physical activity in your life and stick to it:

1. Shallow reasons for exercise (better appearance, status, etc.) can help get you motivated, but the primary way to keep your motivation high in the long run is to do it because it increases the quality of your life. The intrinsic reasons to exercise – self-improvement, enjoyment, challenging yourself, and self-expression – will always take you farther than just wanting to have a nice body.

2. Don't underestimate the power of fun, because in the long run, it's the only way to get plenty of exercise each week and still look forward to the next one.

Boring fitness classes, sports that don't fit your strengths and preferences, and exercises you're doing because you're "supposed to do them" are useless for the proper habit formation. Start your exercise journey by figuring out what fires you up and vow to become great at it – while enjoying yourself, not sweating your guts out and hating every single moment of it.

3. You aren't saving time by not exercising. If anything, you're engaging in a bad trade-off of saving, say, 30 minutes a day just to lose an additional hour of productivity and increase the risk of time-consuming health disorders. Making excuses not to exercise due to a lack of time is also a decision – a decision to say no to your health and suffer the consequences later on.

4. Recovery and the smart approach to exercise in general is a crucial part of every routine for someone who engages in physical activity a few times a week. Don't expect to always have high energy and live a pain-free life if you neglect proper warm-up, getting enough sleep, eating a healthy diet, paying attention to the proper technique while exercising, and giving your body other opportunities to recharge.

5. Don't sweat it. If you associate exercise with something difficult to introduce, you'll always think about it in terms of willpower and self-discipline. Instead, take the "work" out of your workouts and make it about play, self-discovery, and self-expression.

Last, but most definitely not least, please keep in mind that my book can only give you some tools and guidelines on how to start exercising. The second part of the equation – you taking action on it – is the only thing that can change your life.

In the past, I used to read dozens of books only to finish one and start the next one with no consideration for the practical advice the author recommended in the book. It was only when I switched my modus operandi to acting upon advice that non-fiction books, articles, and other resources of all kinds started working for me.

Will this book work for you? The answer now lies in your hands.

Download another Book for Free

I want to thank you for buying my book and offer you another book (just as valuable as this book), *Grit: How to Keep Going When You Want to Give Up*, completely free.

Visit the link below to receive it:

http://www.profoundselfimprovement.com/selfdi sciplinetoexercise

In *Grit*, I'll share with you exactly how to stick to your goals according to peak performers and science.

In addition to getting *Grit*, you'll also have an opportunity to get my new books for free, enter giveaways, and receive other valuable emails from me.

Again, here's the link to sign up:

http://www.profoundselfimprovement.com/selfdi sciplinetoexercise

Could You Help?

I'd love to hear your opinion about my book. In the world of book publishing, there are few things more valuable than honest reviews from a wide variety of readers.

Your review will help other readers find out whether my book is for them. It will also help me reach more readers by increasing the visibility of my book.

About Martin Meadows

Martin Meadows is the pen name of an author who has dedicated his life to personal growth. He constantly reinvents himself by making drastic changes in his life.

Over the years, he has regularly fasted for over 40 hours, taught himself two foreign languages, lost over 30 pounds in 12 weeks, ran several businesses in various industries, took ice-cold showers and baths, lived on a small tropical island in a foreign country for several months, and wrote a 400-page long novel's worth of short stories in one month.

Yet, self-torture is not his passion. Martin likes to test his boundaries to discover how far his comfort zone goes.

His findings (based both on his personal experience and scientific studies) help him improve his life. If you're interested in pushing your limits and learning how to become the best version of yourself, you'll love Martin's works.

You can read his books here:

http://www.amazon.com/author/martinmeadows.

[i] Oaten, M.; Cheng, K. (2006); "Longitudinal gains in self-regulation from regular physical exercise." *British Journal of Health Psychology* 11 (4): 717–733. DOI: 10.1348/135910706X96481.

[ii] Summary Health Statistics: National Health Interview Survey (2014); "Table A-14a. Age-adjusted percent distributions (with standard errors) of participation in leisure-time aerobic and muscle-strengthening activities that meet the 2008 federal physical activity guidelines among adults aged 18 and over, by selected characteristics: United States, 2014."

[iii] Rye, J. A.; Rye, S. L.; Tessaro, I.; Coffindaffer, J. (2009); "Perceived barriers to physical activity according to stage of change and body mass index in the west Virginia Wisewoman population." *Women's Health Issues* 19 (2): 126–134. DOI: 10.1016/j.whi.2009.01.003.

[iv] *Ryan, R. M.; Deci, E. L. (2000). "Self-determination theory and the facilitation of intrinsic motivation, social development, and well-being". American Psychologist 55 (1): 68–78. DOI: 10.1037/0003-066X.55.1.68.*

[v] Gagné, M.; Deci, E. L. (2005) "Self-determination theory and work motivation." *Journal of Organizational Behavior* 26 (4): 331–362. DOI: 10.1002/job.322

[vi] Cho, Y. J.; Perry, J. L. (2012) "Intrinsic Motivation and Employee Attitudes: Role of Managerial Trustworthiness, Goal Directedness, and Extrinsic Reward Expectancy." *Review of Public Personnel Administration* 32 (4): 382–406. DOI: 10.1177/0734371X11421495

[vii] Crane, M. M.; Tate, D. F.; Finkelstein, E. A.; Linnan, L. A. (2012); "Motivation for Participating in a Weight Loss Program and Financial Incentives: An Analysis from a Randomized Trial". *Journal of Obesity* 2012: 290589. DOI: 10.1155/2012/290589.

[viii] *Ryan, R. M.; Deci, E. L. (2000). "Self-determination theory and the facilitation of intrinsic motivation, social development, and well-being". American Psychologist 55 (1): 68–78. DOI: 10.1037/0003-066X.55.1.68.*

153

[ix] Ryan, R. M.; Frederick, C. M.; Lepes, D.; Rubio, N.; Sheldon, K. M. (1997); "Intrinsic Motivation and Exercise Adherence." *International Journal of Sport Psychology* 28: 335–354.

[x] Grant, A. (2013). *Give and Take: A Revolutionary Approach to Success*. Viking Press.

[xi] Grant, A. M., & Berg, J. M. (2011). Prosocial motivation at work: When, why, and how making a difference makes a difference. In K. Cameron & G. Spreitzer (Eds.), *The Oxford Handbook of Positive Organizational Scholarship*. New York: Oxford University Press.

[xii] Uysal, M.; Jurowski, C. (1994). "Testing the push and pull factors". *Annals of Tourism Research* 21 (4): 844–846. DOI: 10.1016/0160-7383(94)90091-4.

[xiii] Irwin, B. C.; Scorniaenchi, J.; Kerr, N. L.; Eisenmann, J. C.; Feltz, D. L. (2012); "Aerobic exercise is promoted when individual performance affects the group: a test of the Kohler motivation gain effect." *Annals of Behavioral Medicine: a Publication of the Society of Behavioral Medicine* 44 (2): 151–9. DOI: 10.1007/s12160-012-9367-4.

[xiv] Feltz, D. L.; Irwin, B. C.; Kerr, N. (2012); "Two-player partnered exergame for obesity prevention: using discrepancy in players' abilities as a strategy to motivate physical activity." *Journal of Diabetes Science and Technology* 6 (4): 820–7. DOI: 10.1177/193229681200600413.

[xv] Duhigg, C. (2012). *The Power of Habit: Why We Do What We Do, and How to Change*. Cornerstone Digital.

[xvi] Clear, J. The 3 R's of Habit Change: How To Start New Habits That Actually Stick. Retrieved December 10, 2015, from http://jamesclear.com/three-steps-habit-change

[xvii] Babauta, L. The Four Habits that Form Habits. Retrieved December 10, 2015, from http://zenhabits.net/habitses/

[xviii] Booth, F. W., Roberts, C. K., Laye, M. J. (2012); "Lack of exercise is a major cause of chronic diseases." *Comprehensive Physiology* 2 (2): 1143–211. DOI: 10.1002/cphy.c110025.

[xix] I-Min, L.; Shiroma, E. J.; Lobelo, F.; Puska, P.; Blair, S. N.; Katzmarzyk, P. T. (2012); "Effect of physical inactivity on

major non-communicable diseases worldwide: an analysis of burden of disease and life expectancy." *The Lancet.* Published online July 18 2012. DOI: 10.1016/S0140-6736(12)61031-9.
[xx] Ekelund, U. et al (2015); "Activity and all-cause mortality across levels of overall and abdominal adiposity in European men and women: the European Prospective Investigation into Cancer and Nutrition Study (EPIC)." *American Journal of Clinical Nutrition* 101 (3): 613–621. DOI: 10.3945/ajcn.114.100065
[xxi] Health.gov, Physical Activity Guidelines, Retrieved December 15, 2015, from http://health.gov/paguidelines/guidelines/adults.aspx
[xxii] Craft, L. L; Perna, F. M. (2004); "The benefits of exercise for the clinically depressed." *Primary Care Companion to the Journal of Clinical Psychiatry* 6 (3): 104–111.
[xxiii] Broman-Fulks, J. J.; Berman, M. E.; Rabian, B. A.; Webster M. J. (2004); "Effects of aerobic exercise on anxiety sensitivity." *Behaviour Research and Therapy* 42 (2): 125–136. DOI: 10.1016/S0005-7967(03)00103-7.
[xxiv] Carek, P. J.; Laibstain, S. E.; Carek, S. M. (2011); "Exercise for the treatment of depression and anxiety." *International Journal of Psychiatry in Medicine* 41 (1): 15–28. DOI: 10.2190/PM.41.1.c.
[xxv] Elavsky, S. (2010); "Longitudinal examination of the exercise and self-esteem model in middle-aged women." *Journal of Sport & Exercise Psychology* 32 (6): 862–80.
[xxvi] Pretty, J., Peacock, J., Sellens, M., Griffin, M. (2005); "The mental and physical health outcomes of green exercise." *International Journal of Environmental Health Research* 15 (5): 319–37. DOI: 10.1080/09603120500155963.
[xxvii] Griffin, É. W.; Mullally, S.; Foley, C.; Warmington, S. A.; O'Mara S. M.; Kelly A. M. (2011); "Aerobic exercise improves hippocampal function and increases BDNF in the serum of young adult males." *Physiology and Behavior* 104 (5): 934–41. DOI: 10.1016/j.physbeh.2011.06.005.

[xxviii] Intlekofer, K. A.; Cotman, C. W. (2013); "Exercise counteracts declining hippocampal function in aging and Alzheimer's disease." *Neurobiology of disease* 57: 47–55. DOI: 10.1016/j.nbd.2012.06.011.

[xxix] von Thiele Schwarz, U.; Hasson, H. (2011); "Employee self-rated productivity and objective organizational production levels: effects of worksite health interventions involving reduced work hours and physical exercise." *Journal of Occupational and Environmental Medicin*e 53 (8): 838–44. DOI: 10.1097/JOM.0b013e31822589c2.

[xxx] Puetz, T. W.; Flowers, S. S.; O'Connor, P. J. (2008); "A randomized controlled trial of the effect of aerobic exercise training on feelings of energy and fatigue in sedentary young adults with persistent fatigue." *Psychotherapy and Psychosomatics* 77 (3): 167–74. DOI: 10.1159/000116610.

[xxxi] Steinberg, H.; Sykes, E. A.; Moss, T.; Lowery, S.; LeBoutillier, N.; Dewey, A. (1997); "Exercise enhances creativity independently of mood." *British Journal of Sports Medicine* 31: 240–245. DOI: 10.1136/bjsm.31.3.240.

[xxxii] Youngstedt, S. D. (2005); "Effects of exercise on sleep." *Clinics in sports medicine* 24 (2): 355–65. DOI: 10.1016/j.csm.2004.12.003.

[xxxiii] Gonzalez, J. T.; Veaseya, R. C.; Rumbold, P. L. S.; Stevenson, E. J. (2013); "Breakfast and exercise contingently affect postprandial metabolism and energy balance in physically active males." *British Journal of Nutrition* 110 (4): 721–732. DOI: 10.1017/S0007114512005582.

[xxxiv] Ariyoshi, M. et al. (1996); "Efficacy of aquatic exercises for patients with low-back pain." *The Kurume Medical Journal* 46 (2): 91–96. DOI: 10.2739/kurumemedj.46.91

[xxxv] Waller, B.; Lambeck, J.; Daly, D. (2009); "Therapeutic aquatic exercise in the treatment of low back pain: A systematic review." *Clinical Rehabilitation* 23 (1): 3–14. DOI: 10.1177/0269215508097856.

[xxxvi] Suzuki S. (2011), *Zen Mind, Beginner's Mind*, Shambhala Publications; Anv edition.

xxxvii Trapani, G. (2007, July 24). Jerry Seinfeld's Productivity Secret. Retrieved December 21, 2015, from http://lifehacker.com/281626/jerry-seinfelds-productivity-secret

xxxviii Johnson, F.; Wardle, J. (2011); "The association between weight loss and engagement with a web-based food and exercise diary in a commercial weight loss programme: a retrospective analysis." *International Journal of Behavioral Nutrition and Physical Activity* 8: 83. DOI: 10.1186/1479-5868-8-83.

xxxix Karageorghis, C. I.; Priest, D. L. (2012); "Music in the exercise domain: a review and synthesis (Part I)." *International Review of Sport and Exercise Psychology* 5 (1): 44–66. DOI: 10.1080/1750984X.2011.631026.

xl Arkes, H. R.; Blumer, C. (1985); "The psychology of sunk costs." *Organizational Behavior and Human Decision Processes* 35: 124–140. DOI: 10.1016/0749-5978(85)90049-4.

xli Frappier, J.; Toupin, I.; Levy, J. L.; Aubertin-Leheudre, M.; Karelis, A. D. (2013); "Energy Expenditure during Sexual Activity in Young Healthy Couples." *PLOS ONE* 8 (10): e79342. DOI: 10.1371/journal.pone.0079342.

xlii Schoenfeld, B.; Contreras, B. (2013); "Is Postexercise Muscle Soreness a Valid Indicator of Muscular Adaptations?" *Strength & Conditioning Journal* 35 (5): 16–21. DOI: 10.1519/SSC.0b013e3182a61820.

xliii Cheatham, S. W.; Kolber, M. J.; Cain, M.; Lee, M. (2015); "The effects of self-myofascial release using a foam roll or roller massager on joint range of motion, muscle recovery, and performance: a systematic review." International Journal of Sports Physical Therapy 10 (6): 827–838. PMCID: PMC4637917.

xliv Beardsley, C.; Škarabot, J. (2015); "Effects of self-myofascial release: A systematic review." *Journal of Bodywork and Movement Therapies* 19 (4): 747–758. DOI: 10.1016/j.jbmt.2015.08.007.

xlv Pearcey, E.; Bradbury-Squires, D. J.; Kawamoto, J. E.; Drinkwater, E. J.; Behm, D. G., Button, D. C. (2015); "Foam Rolling for Delayed-Onset Muscle Soreness and Recovery of

157

Dynamic Performance Measures." *Journal of Athletic Training* 50 (1): 5–13. DOI: 10.4085/1062-6050-50.1.01.

[xlvi] Hillbert, J. E.; Sforzo, G. A.; Swensen, T. (2003); "The effects of massage on delayed onset muscle soreness." *British Journal of Sports Medicine* 37: 72–75. DOI: 10.1136/bjsm.37.1.72.

[xlvii] Zainuddin, Z.; Newton, M.; Sacco, P.; Nosaka, K. (2005); "Effects of Massage on Delayed-Onset Muscle Soreness, Swelling, and Recovery of Muscle Function." *Journal of Athletic Training* 40 (3): 174–180. PMCID: PMC1250256.

[xlviii] Weerapong, P.; Hume, P.A.; Kolt, G. S. (2005); "The mechanisms of massage and effects on performance, muscle recovery and injury prevention." *Sports Medicine* 35 (3): 235–256. DOI: 10.2165/00007256-200535030-00004.

[xlix] Nelson, N. (2013); "Delayed onset muscle soreness: Is massage effective?" *Journal of bodywork and movement therapies* 17 (4): 475–482. DOI: 10.1016/j.jbmt.2013.03.002.

[l] Hurley, C. F.; Hatfield, D. L.; Riebe, D. A. (2013); "The effect of caffeine ingestion on delayed onset muscle soreness." *Journal of Strength and Conditioning Research* 27 (11): 3101–3109. DOI: 0.1519/JSC.0b013e3182a99477.

[li] Kraemer, W. J. et al (2006); "The effects of amino acid supplementation on hormonal responses to resistance training overreaching." *Metabolism* 55 (3): 282–291. DOI/10.1016/j.metabol.2005.08.023

[lii] Shimomura, J. et al (2010); "Branched-chain amino acid supplementation before squat exercise and delayed-onset muscle soreness." *International Journal Of Sport Nutrition And Exercise Metabolism* 20 (3): 236–244. PMID: 20601741.

[liii] Dekkers, J. C.; van Doornen, L. J.; Kemper, H. C. (1996); "The role of antioxidant vitamins and enzymes in the prevention of exercise-induced muscle damage." *Sports Medicine* 21 (3): 213–238. DOI: 10.2165/00007256-199621030-00005.

[liv] Connolly, D. A.; McHugh, M. P.; Padilla-Zakour, O. I.; Carlson, L.; Sayers, S. P. (2006); "Efficacy of a tart cherry juice blend in preventing the symptoms of muscle damage." *British*

Journal of Sports Medicine 40 (8): 679–683. DOI: 10.1136/bjsm.2005.025429.

[lv] Bowtell, J. L.; Sumners, D. P.; Dyer, A.; Fox, P.; Mileva, K. N. (2011); "Montmorency cherry juice reduces muscle damage caused by intensive strength exercise." *Medicine and Science in Sports and Exercise* 43 (8): 1544–51. DOI: 10.1249/MSS.0b013e31820e5adc.

[lvi] Howatson, G.; McHugh, M. P.; Hill, J. A.; Brouner, J.; Jewell, A. P.; van Someren, K. A.; Shave, R. E.; Howatson, S. A. (2010); "Influence of tart cherry juice on indices of recovery following marathon running." *Scandinavian Journal of Medicine and Science in Sports* 20 (6): 843–52. DOI: 10.1111/j.1600-0838.2009.01005.x.

[lvii] Kuehl, K. S.; Perrier, E. T.; Elliot, D. L.; Chesnutt, J. C. (2010); "Efficacy of tart cherry juice in reducing muscle pain during running: a randomized controlled trial." *Journal of the International Society of Sports Nutrition* 7 (7): 17. DOI: 10.1186/1550-2783-7-17.

[lviii] Woods, K.; Bishop, P.; Jones, E. (2007); "Warm-up and stretching in the prevention of muscular injury." *Sports Medicine* 37 (12): 1089–99. DOI: 10.2165/00007256-200838100-00006.

[lix] Fradkin, A. J.; Zazryn, T. R.; Smoliga, J. M. (2010); "Effects of warming-up on physical performance: a systematic review with meta-analysis." *Journal of Strength and Conditioning Research* 24 (1): 140–148. DOI: 10.1519/JSC.0b013e3181c643a0.

[lx] Gergley, J. C. (2013); "Acute effect of passive static stretching on lower-body strength in moderately trained men." *Journal of Strength and Conditioning Research* 27 (4): 973–977. DOI: 10.1519/JSC.0b013e318260b7ce.

[lxi] Simic, L.; Sarabon, N.; Markovic, G. (2013); "Does pre-exercise static stretching inhibit maximal muscular performance? A meta-analytical review." *Scandinavian Journal of Medicine & Science in Sports* 23 (2): 131–148. DOI: 10.1111/j.1600-0838.2012.01444.x.

159

[lxii] Herbert, R. D.; Noronha de M.; Kamper, S. J. (2011); "Stretching to prevent or reduce muscle soreness after exercise." *The Cochrane Database of Systematic Reviews* 6 (7): CD004577. DOI: 10.1002/14651858.

[lxiii] Tsatsouline, P. (2008, December 18). Pavel: 80/20 Powerlifting and How to Add 110 Pounds to Your Lifts. Retrieved 2016, from http://www.fourhourworkweek.com/blog/2008/12/18/pavel-8020-powerlifting-and-how-to-add-110-pounds-to-your-lifts/.

[lxiv] Herman, S. L.; Smith, D. T. (2008); "Four-Week Dynamic Stretching Warm-up Intervention Elicits Longer-Term Performance Benefits." *Journal of Strength & Conditioning Research* 22 (4): 1286–1297. DOI: 10.1519/JSC.0b013e318173da50.

[lxv] Khamwong, P.; Paungmali, A.; Pirunsan, U.; Joseph, L. (2015); "Prophylactic Effects of Sauna on Delayed-Onset Muscle Soreness of the Wrist Extensors." *Asian Journal of Sports Medicine* 6 (2): e25549. DOI: 10.5812/asjsm.6(2)2015.25549.

[lxvi] MacMillan, A. (2015, April 8). Do Saunas Help or Hurt Sore Muscles? Retrieved January 4, 2016, from http://www.outsideonline.com/1966201/do-saunas-help-or-hurt-sore-muscles

[lxvii] Cohen, D. A.; Wang, W.; Wyatt, J. K.; Kronauer, R. E.; Dijk, D.; Czeisler, C. A.; Klerman, E. B. (2010); "Uncovering residual effects of chronic sleep loss on human performance." *Science Translational Medicine* 2 (14): 14ra3. DOI: 10.1126/scitranslmed.3000458.

[lxviii] Lim, J.; Dinges, D. F. (2010); "A Meta-Analysis of the Impact of Short-Term Sleep Deprivation on Cognitive Variables." *Psychological Bulletin* 136 (3): 375–389. DOI: 10.1037/a0018883.

[lxix] Pilcher, J. J.; Huffcutt, A. I. (1996); "Effects of sleep deprivation on performance: a meta-analysis." *Sleep* 19 (4): 318–326.

[lxx] Halson, S. L. (2014); "Sleep in Elite Athletes and Nutritional Interventions to Enhance Sleep." *Sports Medicine* 44 (1): 13–23. DOI: 10.1007/s40279-014-0147-0.

[lxxi] Pejovic, S.; Basta, M.; Vgontzas, A. N.; Kritikou, I.; Shaffer, M. L.; Tsaoussoglou, M.; Stiffler, D.; Stefanakis, Z.; Bixler, E. O.; Chrousos, G. P. (2013); "Effects of recovery sleep after one work week of mild sleep restriction on interleukin-6 and cortisol secretion and daytime sleepiness and performance." *American Journal of Physiology – Endocrinology and Metabolism* 305 (7): E890-6. DOI: 10.1152/ajpendo.00301.2013.

[lxxii] Lautenbacher, S.; Kundermann, B.; Krieg, J. C. (2006); "Sleep deprivation and pain perception." *Sleep Medicine Reviews* 10 (5): 357–369. DOI: 10.1016/j.smrv.2005.08.001.

[lxxiii] Koltyn, K. F. (2000); "Analgesia following exercise: a review." *Sports Medicine* 29 (2): 85–98. DOI: 10.2165/00007256-200029020-00002.

[lxxiv] Yamane, M.; Ohnishi, N.; Matsumoto, T. (2015); "Does Regular Post-exercise Cold Application Attenuate Trained Muscle Adaptation?" *International Journal of Sports Medicine* 36 (8): 647–653. DOI: 10.1055/s-0034-1398652.

[lxxv] Glasgow, P. D.; Ferris, R.; Bleakley, C. M. (2013); "Cold water immersion in the management of delayed-onset muscle soreness: Is dose important? A randomised controlled trial." *Physical Therapy in Sport* 15 (4): 228–233. DOI: 10.1016/j.ptsp.2014.01.002.

[lxxvi] Pournot, H.; Bieuzen, F.; Louis, J.; Fillard, J. R.; Barbiche, E.; Hausswirth C. (2011); "Time-Course of Changes in Inflammatory Response after Whole-Body Cryotherapy Multi Exposures following Severe Exercise." PLOS ONE 6 (7): e22748. DOI: 10.1371/journal.pone.0022748.

[lxxvii] Despain, D. (2015, April 30). A Recovery Ice Bath Isn't (Always) Such a Good Idea. Retrieved December 31, 2015, from http://www.outsideonline.com/1971446/recovery-ice-bath-isnt-always-such-good-idea

161

[lxxviii] Lateef, F. (2010); "Post exercise ice water immersion: Is it a form of active recovery?" *Journal of Emergencies, Trauma and Shock* 3 (3): 302. DOI: 10.4103/0974-2700.66570.

[lxxix] Despain, D. (2015, April 30). A Recovery Ice Bath Isn't (Always) Such a Good Idea. Retrieved December 31, 2015, from http://www.outsideonline.com/1971446/recovery-ice-bath-isnt-always-such-good-idea

[lxxx] Feruggia, J. (2011, November 12). Jason Ferruggia's Renegade Fitness. Retrieved December 30, 2015, from http://jasonferruggia.com/my-1-most-bestest-baddest-training-secret-ever/

[lxxxi] Berhkan, M. (2011, September 27). Fuckarounditis | Intermittent fasting diet for fat loss, muscle gain and health. Retrieved January 6, 2016, from http://www.leangains.com/2011/09/fuckarounditis.html

[lxxxii] Bandura, A. (1977); "Self-efficacy: Toward a unifying theory of behavioral change." *Psychological Review* 84 (2): 191–215. DOI: 10.1037/0033-295X.84.2.191.

[lxxxiii] McNatt, D. B.; Judge, T. A. (2004); "Boundary Conditions of the Galatea Effect: A Field Experiment and Constructive Replication." *Academy of Management Journal* 47 (4): 550–565. DOI: 10.2307/20159601.

Printed in Great Britain
by Amazon

58884636R00097